An Insider's Guide to Working with Healthcare Consultants

T0206452

ACHE Management Series

An
Insider's
Guide to
Working
with
Healthcare
Consultants

Andrew C. Agwunobi

Foreword by
Paul Osborne

ACHE Management Series

Found an error or typo? We want to know! Please e-mail it to hapbooks@ache.org, mentioning the book's title and putting "Book Error" in the subject line.

For photocopying and copyright information, please contact Copyright Clearance Center at www.copyright.com or (978) 750-8400.

Acquisitions editor: Janet Davis; Project manager: Joseph R. Pixler; Cover designer: Brad Norr; Layout: PerfecType

Health Administration Press
A division of the Foundation of the American
  College of Healthcare Executives
300 S. Riverside Plaza
Suite 1900
Chicago, IL 60606-6698
(312) 424-2800

To my mother and father

Contents

Foreword

EMBARKING ON A multimillion-dollar consulting engagement is a difficult task for even the most seasoned CEO. Done correctly, it can be a transformative experience that sets an organization on the path to success. If not, it can be a major disruptive experience that leaves a negative impact.

Andy Agwunobi's book is a must-read for both new and seasoned executives who are contemplating whether to bring in consultants. This doctor's advice is spot-on, and it will greatly increase the odds of having a positive consulting outcome.

I have been a healthcare consultant for more than 25 years, working for some of the largest healthcare consulting firms in the world before joining Berkeley Research Group (BRG) to start a healthcare performance improvement (HPI) practice. Andy was a client of mine, and he was one of the best CEOs I worked with.

Our relationship goes back more than 15 years. We met when Andy was a young physician CEO taking over the helm at a financially struggling public hospital. The organization was distressed and needed to cut costs drastically. Realizing the need for outside expert assistance, Andy and his executive team interviewed multiple consulting firms. They selected the firm I was working for at the time, and I was assigned to run the fast-paced engagement. It required difficult decisions to achieve a quick turnaround, and helped set the organization on a stable footing to implement a long-term strategic plan. Andy and I continued to work together as I moved to other consulting firms and he moved to lead other health systems. In

2011, I was thrilled when he joined me on the consulting side to help build the HPI practice at BRG.

Andy's unique experience and insight, both as a CEO who guides consulting engagements and a consultant responsible for selling and leading consulting engagements, is evident in this book. Rarely does a longtime CEO make the transition to consulting—an unglamorous lifestyle of extensive travel, sales goals, and the responsibility (without any direct authority) of convincing clients to implement your recommendations. Andy was extremely effective in the transition, and a key contributor to building BRG's HPI practice from a start-up to one of the largest in the country. He gained perspective from successes on both sides.

With this book, he will help other CEOs make the right decisions about when to hire the best consultants, and then how to negotiate fees, establish communications, build infrastructure, and manage an engagement to achieve the satisfying result of a truly transformational consulting experience.

Paul Osborne
Managing Director, Berkeley Research Group

Preface

IN 2011, AT 45 years of age, I went from being a career hospital CEO (the regional CEO for five hospitals in Washington State) to being a managing director in the healthcare performance improvement practice of a national consulting firm. Becoming a consultant was a shock. I traded my plush office with private bathroom for packed airports, uncomfortable plane seats, tired hotels, and dilapidated "team rooms" in hospital basements. I swapped the omnipresent support of a high-performing executive assistant for my own weak skills in scheduling and logistics. (I will leave for another day the tales of my debacles, such as finding myself outside an old mattress factory in Connecticut when I should have been delivering a presentation two hours away at a seaside resort in Providence, Rhode Island.) I gave up "you are the boss" status for "the client is the boss" realities, even when the client had a fraction of my experience.

Today, I am back to leading hospitals, but I would not trade the consulting experience for anything. I am a much better, humbler leader for the almost five years I spent as a consultant. The experience shattered my belief that, after more than a decade managing hospitals, I had learned almost all there was to know about improving them. My consulting colleagues showed me how to use data, interviews, and direct observation to analyze a hospital system—much as a physician might diagnose a patient—and then implement the fixes.

I wrote this book not to teach hospital leaders how to become consultants but rather to teach hospital leaders how to best use consultants. As I settled into my new consulting role and began to interact with clients, I thought I was looking into a mirror. I realized that many hospital leaders, like me in my previous life, knew little about consultants or the consulting world. This unfamiliarity clearly detracted from the leaders' ability to optimize consulting engagements. Many times, I wished I could pull them aside and say, "You are focusing on the wrong issue" or "You are asking the wrong question" or even "If you don't follow this advice, you may lose your job." Unfortunately, the imbalance of power between consultant and leader, the lack of a close relationship, and sometimes the mistrust of consultants either precluded this forthrightness or prevented its acceptance.

I wrote this book for leaders who are thinking about hiring consultants or who want to ensure the success of consultants they have already hired. This is the book I wish I had when I started my career as a hospital CEO. In those days, before I began the demystifying experience of becoming a consultant, I hired consultants as infrequently as possible. Today, I am much quicker to hire consultants and less anxious when I do. My hope is that this book will give you the same confidence I acquired, but without having to spend five years on a plane.

Andy
Andrew C. Agwunobi, MD

Acknowledgments

THIS BOOK IS the result of a chapter in my life in which a wonderful organization, Berkeley Research Group (BRG), embraced me and showed me how to bring value to others through consulting. My special thanks to David J. Teece, chairman and principal executive officer of BRG, and to Paul Osborne, managing director of BRG's healthcare performance improvement practice. Paul introduced me to the world of consulting, advised me on this book, and facilitated the consultants survey that I used in doing research for this book. My thanks also to the staff at Health Administration Press, notably Janet Davis and, of course, Joseph Pixler, who for the second time has made the editing process as painless and effective as possible. Finally, my thanks to Elizabeth—my wife, my teammate, and my best friend.

CHAPTER 1

The Value of This Book

CONSULTANT'S TIP

Be engaged. A typical project can last 12 months, and staying engaged for the duration is critical. This is not the consulting firm's project; it is the client's project. The client needs to be involved in each facet to drive change and ensure sustainability. Executive engagement is particularly important for workforce consulting. Department managers will take their lead from their director, who in turn will take their lead from their vice president. If that vice president is not a driving force for the project, success will be limited because the project will not be a priority.

—*Director, labor consulting*

THIS BOOK IS a guide for hospital and health systems executives who are considering the need for a consulting engagement. If you are like most hospital leaders, you dislike the idea of paying for an expensive consulting project. There is the anxiety that you may not really need consultants; and if you do need them, they may not give you good value for your money. You feel at a disadvantage because you are unfamiliar with the consulting industry. You have no way of knowing whether the claims a consulting firm makes are true or a quoted price is fair. You also dread the sales pitch because you fear you will be pressured into paying too much and buying all sorts of unneeded extras. Finally, you are scared of the damage a catastrophic engagement could do to your organization and your credibility as a leader.

These are valid concerns. Although most consulting firms are proud of the service they deliver and all live or die by references from satisfied clients, caveat emptor—buyer beware—applies. Management consulting services are not regulated like hospital services. Anybody can be an "expert." And consultants provide even less price transparency than most hospitals offer. Aggravating the information gap for buyers is a common phenomenon of denial: After spending heavily on a widely publicized but unsuccessful consulting engagement, many hospital leaders are loath to admit that their engagement was a disappointment. They may not agree to serve as a consulting firm's reference, of course, but they also may not be inclined to warn the next unsuspecting client.

I wrote this book to decrease discomfort and risk with consulting engagements. My premise is that you the client can determine the success or failure of your consulting project. If you enter it unprepared and disengaged, you will be disappointed. If you educate yourself and take responsibility for ensuring the success of the engagement, you will see transformative results.

Simply put, this book can help you become an expert on the experts, a master of successful engagements. It will educate you on when to hire consultants, how to choose the right consultants, how to lead your engagement to a successful conclusion, and how to ensure that the improvements stick after the consultants leave. In this book, I describe the mindset and culture of consultants, the inner workings of consulting firms, the drivers of successful engagements, the causes of failure, and techniques to maximize the value of your engagement, including how to negotiate prices. Each chapter also includes case studies and tips that I collected from 40 frontline consultants.

There are many different types of business management consulting engagements, such as information technology, marketing, mergers and acquisitions, and strategy. This book focuses on management consulting for hospitals and health systems. However, because management consulting for hospitals encompasses a wide variety of subspecialties and because all consulting engagements share common themes, the lessons here are applicable to almost all types of consulting (even beyond healthcare).

First, a few words to clarify the term "management consulting." Here is a definition that I like, suggested by educator and development consultant Milan Kubr (International Labour Office 2002, p. 4):

> A method of assisting organizations and executives to improve management and business practices, as well as individual and organizational performance. . . . Ideally, the consultant should choose approaches and methods that uncover and help understand both the technical and the human issues involved, and that help the client to act on both of them.

With hospitals, comprehensive performance improvement engagements range broadly. Usually, they aim to strengthen financial performance by improving key areas such as revenue cycle, labor, patient flow, human resources, physician practice management, clinical variation, perioperative services, and nursing. Comprehensive performance improvement comprises subspecialty-consulting engagements typically aimed at improving hospital finances by improving operations.

There are two hallmarks of comprehensive performance improvement engagements for hospitals:

1. They typically are about improving finances even when the immediate focus is on quality or service.

2. Being comprehensive, they simultaneously encompass multiple specialty areas. They need to be comprehensive because only engagements that capture the complexity of hospitals can improve their finances in a sustainable manner. Some engagements target only one area, such as the operating room or the emergency department (ED), but such narrow engagements will reveal the need for broader efforts if the hospital is to achieve deep and lasting change. For example, it is impossible to improve ED throughput without also improving other areas such as the laboratory, imaging department, bed management, and nurse staffing.

CASE 1

A national consulting firm performed a comprehensive performance improvement engagement for a hospital in California. The hospital, "St. John's," was founded in 1900 by reverend sisters; it now has 500 beds, 2,700 employees, and 680 staff physicians. Between 2011 and 2013, the hospital saw a 4.8 percent decline in inpatient admissions with a 6.0 percent increase in less-well-reimbursed outpatient

→

visits. As a result, St. John's had a negative 4.7 percent operating margin by December 2013. The CEO tried various internal fixes, but eventually the hospital's health system leaders asked her to bring in consultants.

The CEO chose a consulting firm that was already working successfully elsewhere in the system. This engagement included a three-month diagnostic assessment phase when five subspecialty consulting teams identified opportunities for financial improvement in their domains, followed by a nine-month implementation phase when the consultants put their recommendations into motion. At the end of the assessment, the teams identified a low-dollar amount that would be relatively easy to achieve, a middle amount that was difficult but attainable, and a high amount achievable only with extreme difficulty. The hospital and consulting firm settled on a middle target of $18.3 million as the financial improvement goal and the basis for a negotiated implementation price that would render an acceptable return on investment (ROI). They also agreed on an incentive payment to motivate the consulting firm to exceed the $18.3 million.

The engagement went very well. By the end of 12 months, the consulting firm had helped the hospital hit its high target. Just as important, the hospital leadership team appreciated that the firm had, throughout the implementation, stayed true to the faith-based hospital's values. Indeed, at the end of the engagement, an initially skeptical hospital executive sent an e-mail to the firm praising the engagement and the consultants as the best he had ever worked with.

LESSONS

1 Wait until the end of an assessment before deciding on the financial target. This way, the consultants can fully assess the financial opportunity. Choosing a financial target beforehand may lead employees and physicians to fear that the consultants will sacrifice quality to hit an unrealistic target.

2 The success of this engagement shows that hiring consultants can be one of the best decisions you make as a leader. Most leaders experience only a few large consulting engagements in their careers and therefore lack the understanding necessary to maximize their chances of having a St John's-type engagement. This book will help you achieve that depth of understanding.

3 Although this engagement turned out well, it is generally not a good idea for a CEO to wait so long that a board or regional leader directs the CEO to hire a consulting firm. Depending on who actually interviews and hires the firm, this dynamic can create a situation where the consulting firm views the board or regional leader—rather than the hospital CEO—as its boss. In such cases, the assessment may tacitly include determining whether the CEO is part of the problem or part of the solution.

Consider this book your first investment in the success of your large consulting engagement. Consult it constantly on the journey. In fact, read this book before you decide whether to engage consultants because it might persuade you *not* to engage them. Either way, investing just a couple of hours of your time now may save a lot of money for your organization later. If you are embarking on an engagement, read the book and then make it a must-read for the leaders who report to you.

CONSULTANT'S TIP

Clients get their best out of consulting services when (1) they admit they have a problem, communicate this problem to their leaders, and make the case for hiring outside experts to fix the problem, and (2) they agree to be all in—not half in, not 88 percent in—but all in. They do not give up their right to challenge the way we consultants solve a problem, but they should follow our methodologies. And when we state that they have a problem leader who is a barrier to success, they must be willing to make crucial changes. This total commitment should be addressed in the boardroom before a single consultant is deployed.

—Managing consultant, human resources

ENGAGEMENT CHECKLIST

▶ Do you have a bias against consultants?

If you do, then reflect on the reason. If your concerns include those I outlined in the opening paragraph of this chapter, then this book should help calm those fears. If you don't believe consultants are worth the money, consider the fact that pretty much all the hospitals you respect use consultants. It is improbable that they are all wrong. Be open-minded and avoid the mistake of waiting too long to ask for help.

▶ Can you invest the time and attention to detail to manage an engagement?

If not, then appoint a respected and detail-minded executive to serve as the engagement leader from your (the client's) side. You must still stay involved, but your designated executive can give the hands-on leadership that is essential for success.

▶ **Are you worried about what the consultants will find or recommend?**

There is nothing to be concerned about here. When you are a full partner with the consultants and help them implement change, the consultants can be your biggest champions. They can also work with you to avoid changes that could damage the organization.

REFERENCE

International Labour Office. 2002. "Management Consulting in Perspective." In *Management Consulting: A Guide to the Profession,* fourth edition, edited by M. Klubr. Geneva: International Labour Association.

CHAPTER 2

When to Hire Consultants

CONSULTANT'S TIP

View your consultants as employees who are aligned with your goals. Senior leaders should work to ensure that all employees are engaged in the project and accountable for their work.

—*Managing consultant, nonlabor/supply chain practice*

YOU HAVE A problem. Maybe your hospital is hemorrhaging money and you cannot staunch the flow. Or despite your best efforts, your hospital's operating room is stuck in slow motion. Nothing starts on schedule, everything takes too long, and tumbleweed drifts down your corridors during block times. In any event, you are out of ideas, and the board of directors, physicians, or other career-influencing body wants improvement—yesterday! You look around the table at your bleary-eyed senior executive team, and deep down you know they aren't able to fix things. Most are overwhelmed by the current workload, and the few who do have extra capacity wouldn't know how to help you if their lives depended on it. In fact, they are part of the problem. Yes, it is time to consider engaging a consulting firm.

THE COMMITMENT

Don't send out that request for proposals yet. Consulting engagements, particularly comprehensive ones, are expensive, and if they fail, they can traumatize organizations for decades to come. That is why one of the most common refrains consulting firms hear when pitching to clients is "we've done that, and it didn't work." Even successful engagements can be stressful for organizations and generate another common refrain: "My organization is consultant-fatigued." Embarking on a large consulting engagement is an organization-changing decision. You must not only be sure it is the right time to bring in the experts, you must be personally committed to the journey, too.

Commitment starts with overcoming hesitation about hiring outsiders to help fix internal problems. Having mixed feelings about consultants is understandable. Some leaders of distressed organizations view consultants as the shining hope, the commandos. Other leaders mistrust consultants. They fear that these "hired guns" will place lucre before the organization's needs, or they fret that what appears from a distance to be the heroic cavalry will turn out instead to be a horde of hapless Don Quixotes and Sancho Panzas. Truth be told, this fear frequently is tinged with suspicion that some consultants are industry castoffs—that is, of less quality than the clients' own employees. At the other end of the spectrum are leaders who revere consultants so much that they feel insecure in the consultants' presence. These leaders worry that the consultants will find them lacking in knowledge and will label them as part of the problem.

Overcoming hesitancy starts with taking the correct view of what it means to hire consultants. The wrong view is that of buying a used car. This perspective brings the dread of salesman pressure, anxiety about paying too much for what might be a lemon, and self-doubt from a lack of specialized knowledge.

The correct perspective is that you are simply hiring a group of action-oriented, deeply knowledgeable, temporary employees. With this perspective, you will become more confident in hiring and managing consultants.

Once past the hesitancy about the idea of hiring consultants, you must still decide at what point you actually need to hire them.

There are two key reasons (exhibit 2.1) to consider hiring a consulting firm. The first is a lack of bandwidth, meaning there aren't enough people with the time to solve the problem internally. The second key reason is a lack of expertise, meaning no one knows how to solve the problem internally. Of course, you could simply hire permanent employees with both the time and expertise, but by the time you find and hire the right new people, you might run out of time to tackle the problem. Aside from this lack of runway, the degree of risk may make failure to solve the problem unacceptable. Other considerations may include whether your organization has the cash to hire consultants (firms will be leery if you are skirting bankruptcy) and whether you have the support of your boss or board for such an engagement.

Because of the short runway, a decision to engage a consulting firm is a solid commitment. The engagement must work or you will not have time to take alternative action and the plane will crash at takeoff. You must maximize your chances of a successful engagement. The good news is that although for many hospitals recollections of a consulting firm prompt a four-letter word rather than the firm's snappy four-letter acronym name, more hospitals' experiences have been transformational. The aim here is to land in the latter category.

Exhibit 2.1. Decision Tree: When to Hire Consultants

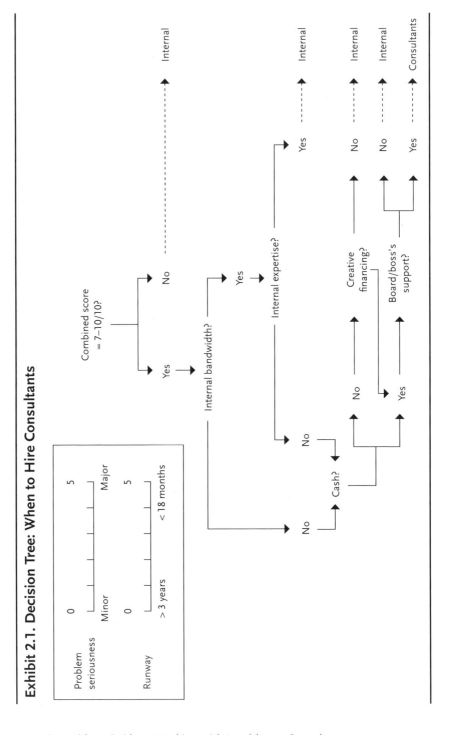

CASE 2

A state-owned academic hospital in the Midwest was losing more than $20 million per year because of a high cost structure, inefficient operations, and the lack of a strategic growth plan.

The hospital leaders faced the question of whether to hire consultants. They knew that at the current rate of losses, they would need to seek a bailout from the state legislature within two years. They desperately wanted to avoid this scenario because seeking such deficit funding would draw widespread criticism from legislators and taxpayers. In addition, the state had financial difficulties of its own, and hospital leaders knew it would deny extra funding. The consulting decision tree in exhibit 2.1 gave the hospital a combined score of 9 out of 10. Clearly, the problem was serious and the runway short.

In terms of bandwidth and expertise, the hospital had enough leaders and employees. Unfortunately, they functioned in silos, thus decreasing the capacity to address systemwide problems in a coordinated manner. In addition, many of the senior leaders lacked the breadth of experience to conduct the needed turnaround.

The leaders decided they needed consulting help. The next challenge was finding a way to pay for it. A few years earlier, the health system had received state funds to renovate several buildings, so it was able to fund the engagement with some of the money it had allocated for preventive maintenance. The board approved the plan, and the health system engaged a national firm to conduct a yearlong comprehensive performance improvement project. The engagement netted $15 million in financial improvement. This happy result averted the need to seek deficit funding for consultants and gave the system time to work on a long-term sustainability plan.

LESSONS

1 Do not wait until you have a crisis to look for consultants. Project your finances for two to three years out, and be realistic (remember, hope is not a strategy) so you can anticipate challenges and hire consultants proactively. Consultants need about a year to implement a large performance improvement engagement, and some of the financial gains will come in the subsequent year. When leadership waits too long to seek help, financial problems may become a crisis midway through a consulting engagement, necessitating massive layoffs or even hospital closure. Consultants can help solve serious financial problems, but they are not magicians.

2 Assess your team to be sure that you do not ask them to fix a problem that lies beyond their capabilities. Some CEOs who know they need consulting help nevertheless will first try to save money by fixing the problems internally. This is prudent if the organization has the necessary bandwidth and experience. If it does not, the result can be can be a costly loss of time that is essential to prevent a crisis.

The following case illustrates a leadership team's decision against embarking on a comprehensive consulting engagement.

CASE 3 An inner-city county children's hospital that was part of a larger public health system (separately licensed) was losing $5 million per year. It also needed $30 million for renovations. No easy financial solutions existed. Leadership had cut costs, but the losses continued. Meanwhile, the

→

parent health system was struggling financially, the county was unwilling to increase support, and philanthropic donations were limited.

Parents also had other choices for children's hospitals, and therefore closure was a real possibility.

The first question was whether to hire consultants. According to the consulting decision tree, the problem was a 5 (major) in seriousness. The runway score, on the other hand, was probably a 2 or 3 because the parent health system could cut costs elsewhere to subsidize the children's hospital for a few more years. Also, closing a hospital, particularly a public children's hospital, was something the leaders knew they could not do precipitously. The combined score was approximately 7, thus passing the first screen for considering a consulting engagement.

The children's hospital was small. Among the leaders of the parent health system and the hospital, enough internal bandwidth existed to implement fixes—if the leaders could identify the solutions. They had tried many strategies over the years, and none worked. They had bandwidth but needed expertise.

The next question for the leaders was whether the parent system had enough cash to pay for a big consulting engagement. The answer was no. The system was already struggling to pay its creditors, so diverting funds to a large consulting engagement was out of the question, particularly for a public institution. In addition, vocal advocates of the hospital feared that consultants might recommend draconian cost cutting or even closure of the children's hospital, and threatened to oppose "any diversion of funds from the care of children to a consulting firm."

→

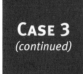

CASE 3
(continued)

Because of the shortage of cash, the system decided not to engage a management consulting firm. Fortunately, the story did not end there. The hospital CEO recognized that although funding was absent for a large performance improvement engagement, the lack of internal expertise made the argument for at least a limited strategy consulting study. He explored creative funding solutions. Eventually, a philanthropic foundation that had donated annually to the children's hospital but was dissatisfied with the lack of a plan for the hospital's sustainability volunteered to pay $50,000 for a strategy study.

The study uncovered important information that helped leaders identify a solution. For example, it revealed the hospital was actually losing $7 million per year, not $5 million (services provided free by the parent health system obscured the true losses). The study also showed that the hospital's small and declining market share across all specialties meant that it would be difficult to reverse these losses. Finally, the study showed that traditional strategic options would be prohibitively expensive. Armed with this information, the health system leaders elected to merge their hospital with a nearby private children's hospital system.

LESSONS

1 When funds are insufficient for a comprehensive consulting study, explore creative approaches to financing. We discuss this more in chapter 6, "Setting the Price."

2 Sometimes a small, inexpensive consulting study can give you the missing information necessary to arrive at definitive solutions. For a small study, the scope should be tightly defined to avoid a broad and superficial Captain Obvious result. In the case of the children's hospital, the engagement focused on elucidating the true financial situation and then recommending potential strategic options.

ENGAGEMENT CHECKLIST

▶ Do you need consultants?

Use the decision tree in exhibit 2.1 to answer this question. If your conclusion is "yes, but I can't afford to hire consultants," think of creative ways to fund at least a limited engagement such as an assessment phase without implementation. A midsize hospital can expect to pay between $150,000 and $350,000 for a three-month organization assessment. If this is too much money, consider a narrowly focused consulting engagement such as a revenue cycle engagement that can yield quick returns.

Do not let the financial problems continue unchecked. As the saying goes, "Hope is not a strategy." Either fix the finances with consultants or fix them with your own employees, but fix them. Otherwise, someone eventually will consider you to be part of the problem. By then, it may be too late to bring in external help. Put another way: Sometimes, you can't afford *not* to hire consultants.

▶ Is your organization ready for consultants?

Be wary about bringing consultants into a dysfunctional and unsupportive culture. A bad culture can kill the best-organized engagement. You will know you have such a culture if your medical staff is disengaged or if your own senior leadership team presents unfounded resistance to bringing in consultants. If your organization is in financial distress, you may lack the time needed to correct the cultural problems before embarking on your consulting engagement. If so, address the cultural tasks in parallel. The fixes might entail launching a physician engagement campaign and coaching or replacing those executives who are working against you. Dropping consultants into a toxic culture and leaving them to fend for themselves guarantees a failed engagement.

▶ Are you ready to invest the personal time and effort that a successful engagement requires?

After hiring the consultants, if your plan is to leave for a long vacation or move onto the next task, you should reconsider hiring consultants. This casual approach won't work with complex engagements. Similar to the implementation of a new electronic health record system, large engagements require full leadership involvement. A hands-off approach greatly increases the risk of failure.

CHAPTER 3

How to Select the Right Consultants

CONSULTANT'S TIP

Organizational leaders and staff should place enthusiasm for improving the organization above personal job satisfaction. They need to take a leap of faith that job satisfaction will improve as the organization improves.

—*Senior managing consultant, physician practice management*

TODAY, A PERSON searching for the best hospital for a particular specialty can turn to the internet or sources such as the *U.S. News & World Report* hospital rankings. For hospital leaders seeking the right management consulting firm, there are few sources to help them choose. One possible option is the *Forbes* "America's best management consulting firms" rankings, but this list doesn't give details such as specific strengths (e.g., revenue cycle consulting), bang-for-the-buck value, or outcomes. *Modern Healthcare* magazine's list of top management consulting firms is another option. Because of a paucity of sources for guidance, many hospitals simply hire firms they have used before or send out requests for proposals (RFPs). For many others, the most common approach is word of mouth, which is highly subjective and frequently leads to poor choices.

THE SELECTION PROCESS

Regardless of where a hospital finds its pool of consulting firms, the final selection process, like the process for hiring employees, typically includes interviews. Well-conducted interviews will reveal the weak firms and lead to the right choice.

To know what makes an interview effective, it helps to understand how consulting firms themselves approach these interviews—or what they refer to as "sales presentations." These are the most important meetings for any consulting firm. One reason is the long sales cycle for hospitals. Six to nine months or even longer may pass from the consulting firm's initial pitch to a senior leader (such as a cold call or conversation at a hospital association meeting) to an engagement, and securing the engagement frequently rests on the consulting firm's performance in a single sales presentation. In addition, depending on the firm's size and current business load, landing that one large engagement can make the difference between hitting or missing year-end financial targets. Finally, these sales presentations are of huge personal importance to the individual consultants. Consulting firms promote and highly compensate senior consultants who are good at originating and securing engagements. For junior consultants, more engagements mean better utilization and job security.

The point is that consultants come to the interview highly motivated to secure the engagement. This buyer's market gives hospitals immense negotiating power but also causes unethical consulting firms to exaggerate their capabilities and experience. Herein lies a key difference between interviewing a person for employment versus interviewing a consulting firm for an engagement. Job candidates bring easily verifiable resumes that document all significant work and education, whereas the consulting firms' resumes (their sales decks) may only include cherry-picked examples of previous clients, the biographies of a small subset of the consultants who will work on the engagement, and assertions of past performance that can be difficult to verify without all relevant details.

Crafting an RFP

Using an RFP to create a short list of interviews can help strengthen the subsequent interview process because good RFPs include requests for specific information about the consulting firms' finances, number of consultants, organizational structure, and so forth. When an RFP requires an authorized officer such as the firm's general counsel to verify the proposal's accuracy, you should be able to trust the answers. Unfortunately, some good consulting firms will give a half-hearted response, or will not respond at all, to an RFP. You may find this surprising, given the earlier point about the importance that consulting firms place on securing engagements. The problem is that RFPs typically include requests for voluminously detailed information that some busy firms consider prohibitively time consuming. In addition, when a hospital sends RFPs to many consulting firms, some may decide the effort to respond is not worth the slim chance of winning an engagement. Finally, consulting firms may believe that a hospital has issued an RFP only for appearances—that is, the hospital wants to appear objective but in truth has already decided which firm will receive the job.

Another downside of RFPs is that they can delay the start of a time-sensitive engagement. This is because in the typical RFP process, several executives and other stakeholders meet over a few weeks to create it, the hospital then gives the consulting firms several weeks or even months to respond, and finally an RFP scoring team takes several additional weeks to review and rank the responses. Add to that the time to schedule and conduct interviews.

Despite the potential problems with RFPs, I recommend this approach. The detailed information they provide is immensely helpful in identifying the right consulting firm. Three ways to mitigate the downsides are:

1. Send the RFP to no more than six to eight firms, and let them know that they are on a short, select list. This will assure the firms that their odds for winning are reasonable.

2.   Limit the number of questions and the word count of responses. This will assure firms that the effort and time to respond will be reasonable.

3.   Allow an RFP response time of no more than three or four weeks. This shortens delays associated with the process. However, reserve flexibility to extend the response time by a few days just in case a good firm misses the deadline.

Whether or not you issue an RFP, you should prepare a list of interview questions to increase objectivity and perceptiveness. Put simply, your goal in conducting interviews is to determine which consulting firm best achieves your aims and is a good fit for your organization. Choosing consulting firms is a bit like choosing a surgeon. You want someone who is qualified, is highly competent in the particular procedure, possesses a good bedside manner, and communicates well.

INTERVIEW QUESTIONS

To identify the right firm for an engagement, interview questions must cover the key topic areas of qualifications, competence, bedside manner, and communication with leadership.

Establishing Qualifications

What can you tell me about your history as a consulting firm?
    This question is akin to a hiring manager asking a job candidate for educational qualifications or a parent asking a pediatric surgeon for the number of surgeries they have performed. Here, the answer will reveal whether the consulting firm is qualified and competent to do your work.
    Unlike employees who must come with stipulated qualifications such as a master's degree, or surgeons with board certification,

consulting firms do not come with any required certification. Their history, however, serves as an effective substitute. A firm that says it can improve a large hospital's supply chain costs, workforce efficiency, physician practice operations, and revenue cycle but has only five employed consultants who came together two years ago to perform patient experience consulting does not have the correct history. On the other hand, a consulting firm with 800 employees, divisions for each of its specialties, and a multiyear history of conducting such engagements does have the correct history.

A firm's list of past clients also is an important part of its history. It is always promising when the list includes impressive clients and clients similar to your organization. If aspects of the firm and its client list don't seem to match (e.g., the firm is small and new but has a long list of major clients), ask whether these were clients of the firm or rather were clients of the individual consultants when they worked at other firms. I once interviewed a small consulting firm that presented a long list of academic medical center clients. Probing deeper, I learned that most of the clients were those of the individual managing directors before they joined this relatively new firm. This is not dishonest, because the individual consultants do the work and their experience is critical. It is not, however, completely forthright because you are interested in the current firm. Therefore, unless the consulting firm declares this nuance proactively, you should raise your guard about the rest of the information it provides. This practice also indicates that the firm must scrape to generate a list of prior clients. One more point: Because there is a clear difference between a whole team working with impressive or similar clients versus individual members working with such clients, you must apply a mental discount to the latter type of list.

This discussion raises an important question: Should you choose a large firm with hundreds of previous clients or choose a small firm? The default position is to go with larger firms, but the correct answer depends on your degree of risk aversion and the budget. If you are risk averse and have plenty of money to spend, then it makes sense to go with a large, established firm that has had many clients similar to your organization. If you are willing to accept more risk (sometimes with a higher return on investment) for a lower cost, a smaller firm could be the right choice for you.

You get experience and bench strength with large firms, but they can be expensive and inflexible in approach, too. Small firms know they may be at a disadvantage in competing with the big guys, so they can play up their lower overhead and greater pricing flexibility—two attributes that allow them to compete on price. Small firms will also be more willing to customize their approach to meeting your needs. A downside is that large engagements may overwhelm them. In addition, because the implementation phase of any engagement is labor intensive, they might conduct a good assessment phase but be incapable of fielding enough consultants to implement their own recommendations. Finally, if you don't like any of their consultants, small firms have limited ability to replace them.

Please introduce the individuals who will be working on our engagement.
It is important to know the credentials of the consultants with whom you will interact daily. The success of your engagement depends on them. Most consulting firms will bring the engagement leader and some team leaders to the interview, but you need to know who will work on your project and who will not. This will prevent any real or perceived bait-and-switch scenario where the seasoned, charismatic consultants who sold you on their firm disappear—replaced by a bunch of juniors as soon as the agreement is signed.

Most consulting firms don't bait and switch, but sometimes clients may not understand that consulting firms approach sales presentations differently than the subsequent engagements. For sales presentations, consulting firms field the best team to secure the sale. There will be overlap, but the sales team is not necessarily the best team for the consulting work. For example, sales teams usually include the consultant who originated the deal (possibly a consultant who has a relationship with someone in the client's leadership team) but may have nothing to do with the actual engagement. Sales teams also typically include at least one of the firm's most charismatic and experienced managing directors, perhaps even the leader of the firm or of the consulting practice in the firm. This "rainmaker" may stay involved after the sale to manage the relationship with the client but may not work directly on the project. The sales team may also include senior subject matter experts such as physicians to advise the teams on specialized issues. These experts work on multiple engagements simultaneously but spend little time on each. In addition, the sales team typically includes someone from the firm's business-development staff.

As mentioned earlier, some members of the sales team will work on the engagement. Specifically, the team usually includes the engagement director (a senior consultant who oversees the project) and a few leaders of specific consulting areas such as patient flow, revenue cycle, and nursing who will work on the project. The consulting firm's ideal is an effective and impressive sales team of reasonable size. A sales team that's too large can make the sales pitch setting potentially chaotic, with consultants talking over or contradicting each other. It can also give prospective clients the impression that the engagement will be pricey. A limited size, however, might mean that up to half of the sales team will not work on your project full time, and some not at all.

To be clear, no matter how charismatic and knowledgeable the consultants on the sales team might be, you do not necessarily want

CONSULTANT'S TIP

A spirit of cooperation and accountability drives overall success. To that point, identify specific initiative owners on your team and engage key stakeholders by setting expectations up front. This ensures better teamwork and follow-through.

—*Senior managing consultant, human resources*

all of them working on your project. A managing director whose hourly rate is high but who hasn't worked on the consulting front lines for years may not bring the best value. Similarly, the consulting firm's sole physician may be important for physician meetings but too expensive for everyday on-site presence. Therefore, rather than requesting that all members of the sales team work on your engagement, ask for the credentials of those—whether present or not—who will work on the engagement, and then make sure they have the requisite experience.

Identifying Competence

Has your firm ever performed this type of consulting engagement? If so, describe the engagements, with outcomes.

Just as with surgeons, the more times a consulting firm has performed your specific type of work, such as reducing staff in a unionized hospital or improving the finances and operations of a multispecialty physician group, the better the firm will be at that work. You should be wary if the firm's answer is something like, "We haven't performed this specific type of engagement, but we have done many that are similar, such as. . . ." Most likely, a surgeon who has performed numerous appendectomies will be more competent at removing your appendix than one who hasn't, even if the latter has performed many other abdominal surgeries. When a consulting firm responds to this question in the affirmative, ask for references from those clients. That way, you can confirm that the projects were indeed the same as yours and that the outcomes were satisfactory.

How will you perform this engagement?

The consulting firm should be able to describe in simple terms what the work will entail, including how long each phase will take.

Do not stop at generic answers such as "we do a data analysis and interviews that enable us to identify the problems." This would be like a surgeon saying he will ask questions and do tests to determine the problem. Yes, but what tests and what questions? Expect the firm to describe specific data they will be looking at and why; the types of questions they will be asking and of whom; and for what reasons. It will quickly become evident whether they plan a fishing or a focused approach. The former is usually a sign of inexperience and sometimes incompetence.

What specific methods will you use to ensure sustainability?

All clients ask this question, but all too often they are satisfied with generic answers such as "we train your staff" or "we leave behind tools." Ask for specifics such as examples of training materials, software tools, and monitoring after the engagement has ended. We address this point further in chapter 13. "Ensuring Sustainability."

Determining Bedside Manner

What will your approach be to my organization as you conduct this engagement?

Your goal here is to determine whether the consulting firm will be able to build trust with your employees. In the interview, good consulting firms will articulate a philosophy, communication approach, and routines to help the organization accept the consultants as an extension of your employees and leadership team. It is helpful to give scenarios. For example: "How will you work to overcome the skepticism of our orthopedic group about reducing the number of device vendors?" The answer will quickly reveal the consulting team's caliber.

Communicating with Leadership

What is your approach to communicating with the organization's senior leaders during the project?

Good consulting firms will communicate frequently and transparently with you and your leadership team. They will also follow your lead on how and when they communicate sensitive information elsewhere, such as to the board and employees. In addition, they will work with you to develop a unified message regarding the engagement.

During the interviews, experienced firms should be able to articulate an organized communication approach that includes standing meetings to keep hospital leaders apprised of the engagement's status.

CASE 4

A hospital in Missouri issued an RFP for a consulting firm to develop a communications and marketing campaign. The hospital leadership interviewed several candidates. On paper, a local firm that understood the hospital's political environment and brand appeared well qualified. However, on the day of the interview, only one person from the firm, a managing director–partner, attended in person. Two other partners participated by phone (one stuck in an airport and the other with unchangeable scheduling conflicts). A few pointed questions revealed the real issue. The firm was extremely small with only a few consultants, mainly the partners themselves, spread over several clients nationwide. The consultants attempted to assure hospital leadership that the small size wouldn't be a problem and insisted that none of their clients had ever felt neglected.

→

CASE 4
(continued)

As the hospital's leadership team probed further, the partners admitted that only the in-person attendee would work day-to-day on the engagement. Because of other client commitments, those on the phone would be involved infrequently and almost never in person. The hospital team suspected that even the consultant involved on a daily basis had limited time to meet the hospital's needs. For example, the firm's PowerPoint presentation for this important meeting appeared rushed. The deck was perfunctory, poorly formatted, and even contained typos. The hospital chose a different, larger firm.

LESSONS

1 Bigger consulting firms are not necessarily better, but tiny firms may struggle to complete a large engagement unless it is their sole client. Most firms will say they can ramp up quickly, and some can. But when you choose such firms, you risk missing deadlines. In addition, because ramping up usually means rapidly hiring consultants who may be unfamiliar with your hospital, the quality of work may suffer.

2 When interviewing a consulting firm, look for signs of problems that may affect your engagement. If the consultants contradict or talk over one another, it can indicate (1) they haven't worked together for long (such as independent consultants who come together infrequently for large engagements), (2) the firm's practices function in silos, or (3) the firm has a dysfunctional culture. The third sign may appear when there is internal competition for the engagement fees or other benefits from originating and securing engagements. In some firms, the practices essentially buy services from each other—say, the revenue cycle practice will buy services from the data analytics practice and the clinical practice. This internal marketplace can lead to competition among practices to control more and more of the engagement's funding. Competition for the credit of having secured an engagement can also occur in firms where senior consultants must generate a multiple of their salaries in sales. When you detect troubling internal dynamics, investigate with pointed questions: Ask how the firm incentivizes its consultants, and how the different practices work together.

3 Presentation materials can tell you a lot. Just as you expect polished resumes from job candidates, you should expect polished presentations from consulting firms. It is a bad sign when a firm creates a presentation that flows poorly or includes typos. Remember: This is the consulting firm at its best. In addition, canned presentations, even when polished, should raise concerns. They may indicate an overstretched firm or one that doesn't adequately value (i.e., need) your business.

REFERENCE CHECKS

Checking references is a critical step in selecting consulting firms, just as it is in hiring permanent employees. Reference checks for firms, however, have the same shortfalls as those for job candidates. No self-respecting consulting firm submits a list of clients who would

---

CONSULTANT'S TIP

Clients should be transparent about other initiatives they are working on that may have an impact on our work.

—*Consultant, revenue cycle*

---

provide anything but glowing references. Sometimes, a reference is glowing because the firm does a good job. Other times, it is glowing because the client (e.g., a hospital CEO) wants to preserve credibility in the face of a hugely expensive failure. You should ask to contact clients beyond the proffered list of references. Consulting firms will worry about this request, but few will refuse.

ENGAGEMENT CHECKLIST

▶ Do you have a process for finding suitable consulting firms?

If your hospital is part of a large system with numerous consulting engagements, the corporate office may already have a list of preapproved consulting firms for you to consider. Many hospitals, however, must find firms on their own. The most thorough approach, as noted in chapter 2, "When to Hire Consultants," is to issue an RFP to a short list of good firms. The *Forbes* and *Modern Healthcare* lists of top consulting firms are good starting points, but visit the firms' websites to understand whether their offerings can meet your needs. Also, these two sources miss good smaller firms, so seek recommendations from other hospitals and your senior executive team, too. If you still can't find enough candidate firms, post your RFP on your website.

▶ Have you set up criteria for screening?

For efficiency, keep the number of consulting firms you interview to no more than eight. This usually requires a screening process, as with discarding job applicants who don't meet basic qualifications. Create screening criteria to ensure you do not eliminate desirable firms and that the selected firms line up with your objectives and your available resources. So if your organization is on the East Coast and you want to keep travel expenses low, you may want to eliminate West Coast firms from consideration.

▶ Have you ensured that your RFP is not onerous?

When writing the RFP, be concise and as specific as possible. Do not ask firms for unnecessary information. Give them enough time to respond, say three to four weeks.

▶ Are you prepared for the interviews?

Prepare well so that you can maximize the benefit of the interviews. In addition to doing your homework with Internet searches for news about the firms, preparation includes giving meeting guidelines to the firms and your interviewers ahead of time. Tell the firms how long the presentation will be as compared to the question and answer (Q&A) portion of the interview, and err on the side of less time for presentation and more for Q&A. Prepare your questions beforehand and distribute them to your colleagues on the interviewing team for their input. Coach your interviewers to focus on asking questions, listening, and rating responses rather than wasting time with long discourses about their own thoughts.

CHAPTER 4

What Consultants Do: Advisory Versus Implementation Firms

> **CONSULTANT'S TIP**
>
> Good medical staff dynamics and physician–C-suite relationships include the willingness of C-suite executives to hold physicians accountable for cost and quality and to walk away from a high-cost, low-quality doctor regardless of their volume.
>
> —*Managing director, clinical consulting*

HOSPITAL LEADERS WILL say that consultants simply look at your watch and tell you the time. The truth is that good consultants scurry across your organization to gather the pieces of the watch, put them all together, and then tell you the time. If the assembled watch is telling the wrong time—as is most likely—the consultants will advise you on how to fix your watch. This is the basic advisory model. The great consultants will go a step further: They will roll up their sleeves and help you fix your watch, for a price. I call these consulting companies *implementation firms*.

To be more specific, *advisory firms* offer clients an assessment (diagnostic) phase that ends in recommendations, whereas *implementation firms* offer an additional phase to execute their recommendations. I place implementation firms a notch above advisory firms because implementation firms structure themselves to be accountable for demonstrating that their recommendations will work. They put their money where their mouths are, so to speak. Only firms that are confident in their competencies take that accountability because they make a sizeable portion of their payment dependent on the client's agreement that the implementation was successful. Specifically, the client must sign an agreement that the consulting firm successfully implemented each recommendation and that the hospital will realize the promised savings or increased revenues. Take, as an example, a situation where labor consultants from an implementation firm recommend new workflows to reduce full-time equivalents without a commensurate reduction in service. For the consultants to get paid, the client's skeptical department directors must confirm in writing that the consultants implemented workflow changes that protected service while generating the promised savings from reduced staffing. It is no surprise that, despite the larger payments associated with implementation engagements (typically a few million dollars versus a few hundred thousand), many consulting firms prefer to make their money on multiple relatively easy advisory engagements rather than a few difficult at-risk implementation engagements.

Here's an illustration of the difficulty associated with implementing recommendations. When working at an implementation firm, I hired an independent contractor to round out a team working on a large financial turnaround project for a hospital. The independent contractor, let's call him "Jake," specialized in improving the efficiency of support staff in physician groups and came highly recommended. The engagement started well. Jake conducted his analysis and identified significant savings from a new staffing model he recommended. That, however, was only the assessment phase. When we entered the implementation phase, Jake fell apart. He didn't know how to help the client get buy-in from the physicians and couldn't put together a risk-based methodology so the client could compensate our firm according to the results. As the implementation dragged on and the client became increasingly dissatisfied, I asked Jake what the problem was. He admitted that, in his two decades of consulting, no firm had ever asked him to implement his recommendations. It was my fault. I hadn't asked the right interview questions, which would have revealed he had only worked for advisory firms. Implementation is hard, and I am not sure who was more relieved when I let him go—Jake or me.

CASE 5

A community hospital in Ohio was concerned about the impact of healthcare reform and declining reimbursements on its healthy operating margin. The hospital issued a request for proposals (RFP) seeking a consulting firm to further strengthen its financial performance. The hospital CEO wanted an assessment, not an implementation engagement. Her rationale was that, over the previous few years, the hospital had sent all managers for Six Sigma training and created a department of black belts (an internal consulting team, of sorts) called the Performance Excellence (PE) department. She believed that after the consultants generated recommendations, the PE department could implement the recommendations less expensively than an external implementation firm could.

The hospital interviewed several firms and, despite not desiring implementation, decided to hire an implementation firm to perform a three-month assessment. The firm identified more than $15 million in improvements but predicted internal implementation would be difficult because many managers and employees were resistant to change. As evidence of this, the PE team expressed skepticism about the feasibility of the consultants' recommendations. The consultants, for their part, felt the PE team lacked the bandwidth, subject matter expertise, and sense of urgency to implement the recommendations without assistance.

→

CASE 5
(continued)

When the consulting firm presented its recommendations, hospital leaders realized the degree of implementation difficulty and the potential rewards of successful implementation. The CEO decided on a hybrid model in which the consultants and the PE team would jointly implement the consultants' recommendations. This model worked well. As the PE team and consultants worked together, they developed mutual trust and respect. In the end, the hospital exceeded its financial improvement targets for the engagement.

LESSONS

1 A sophisticated hospital leadership team will recognize the importance of a credible assessment and will hire a consulting firm that knows how to implement its recommendations. Likewise, seasoned managers and physician leaders will know when a consulting firm's recommendations are impractical, and internal change-management consultants such as PE teams will know when external consultants are lightweights who can't measure up to the demands of a challenge. A benefit of hiring an implementation firm is that its consultants will know whether your employees are capable of implementing change.

2 If you have the equivalent of an internal PE team, give it a central role in planning for and hiring consultants. Assure the team that the consulting engagement is not a criticism of its work or a threat to its role, and include it in the implementation of some initiatives.

3 Even if you think you do not need implementation help, be careful not to preemptively close the door on the possibility. It is a mistake at the beginning of an engagement to broadcast to employees that the consultants are there only for advice, and that they will not participate in implementing their recommendations. You might learn in the assessment that the employees are incapable of the necessary change management without external help.

In practice, the line between implementation and advisory firms can be blurred. This is because few advisory firms will pass on the opportunity to earn more fees by helping a client implement, even if they have to add staff or subcontractors. On the other hand, an implementation firm will happily limit itself to an assessment phase if the client doesn't want to pay for implementation.

Nevertheless, distinguishing one type of firm from the other is important, just as it is important to distinguish a tax expert who offers advice on how to minimize your taxes from a tax expert who offers advice and then prepares and files your taxes. The best way to make the distinction is to ask. Although few consulting firms will say whether they are more comfortable with assessments than implementations, ask them how many of their past five to ten engagements involved implementations. Another good question to ask is, "What is your business model?" or, more bluntly,

CONSULTANT'S TIP

The client should take part in creating deliverables and champion the effort as an organizational initiative, not a consulting firm initiative. Positivity is always a plus!

—*Consultant, revenue cycle*

"Where do you make your money?" Advisory firms make their margins on efficient assessments, generally conducted for a fixed fee; implementation firms make their money in the execution. In fact, they may deliberately lose money conducting an in-depth assessment to ensure success with the subsequent—and more lucrative—implementation.

Knowing whether your organization just needs advice or also needs help in implementing that advice is important. Choosing the former when you need the latter is frequently the cause of an expensive consulting study ending up in a binder on the shelf. In truth, most organizations that choose to engage consultants need implementation help as well as advice. Despite this, many organizations go with advisory engagements, that is, with assessments. They usually do so to limit the consulting fees, the thought being, as in case 5, "if the consultants tell us what to do, my team should be able to implement it." Given the costs of implementation, this approach may sound shrewd, but it ignores the bandwidth problem illustrated by the bleary-eyed senior team in chapter 2, "When to Hire Consultants." It also ignores the fact that at the end of the assessment phase, most consulting firms will tell you what needs to be fixed and perhaps even the steps to fix it, but they will not tell you exactly how to implement those steps.

The following excerpt is from an assessment performed by a respected national consulting firm for a public hospital experiencing millions of dollars in losses per year. The recommendations pertain to establishing incentive-based compensation for physicians and other faculty.

Establish a Comprehensive Compensation Plan. Develop an overall compensation plan that incorporates all the missions and sets aside funding to allow incentives in research and clinical areas. Funding for these plans will be generated by redirecting existing general funds to areas of growth and budgeting the incentive dollars during the budget process. . . . A viable incentive plan to augment base compensation will be a critical part of the plan, including implementing productivity targets for faculty.

This was sound advice. However, anyone—healthcare leader or consultant—who has ever tried to implement a new compensation methodology for physicians knows that going from recommendations to successful implementation is like going from watching the film *Everest* to climbing Everest. Knowing the route to the summit and following expert advice is not enough to get there, or get back home. In this case, the full report, which spanned almost 300 pages, recommended fixes for every major aspect of the health system from the compensation changes to clinical cost savings. Unfortunately, the health system did not request an implementation phase. As a result, it continued to hemorrhage money and yes, several years later, the report sat in a dusty binder on a shelf.

One key advantage to engaging an implementation firm—even when you do not plan to retain the consultants beyond the assessment phase—is that its recommendations are more likely to be realistic, or implementable. Consultants in such firms will avoid recommending infeasible fixes because they realize what it takes to implement difficult change, and they know they might be the ones tasked with delivering their recommendations.

CONSULTANT'S TIP

Keep the organization focused, commit to implementing recommendations, and develop the leadership team on how to manage change effectively.

—*Senior managing consultant, clinical*

ENGAGEMENT CHECKLIST

▶ **Have you decided if your organization needs advisory or implementation help, or both?**

You probably know the answer, but to help with buy-in, ask your direct reports what they think. Overwhelmed managers will usually welcome the implementation help, but they are more likely to do so if they are part of the decision process.

▶ **Are you sure that the consulting firms on your short list are implementation firms?**

You can easily determine this by means of a well-crafted RFP, probing interview questions, and reference checks.

CHAPTER 5

Who Does What and Why

> **CONSULTANT'S TIP**
>
> Clients must stay focused on what they are trying to achieve. This focus can only occur if there is a constant dialogue between the consultant and the client.
>
> —*Managing director, human resources*

GOOD CONSULTING ENGAGEMENTS are partnerships, and partnerships do not work when the character and motivations of the partners are opaque. That's why it's helpful when hospital leaders understand the structure, culture, and incentives of the consulting firms they hire. For example, when they are interviewing potential firms, hospital leaders commonly decide they want the sales team to work on their project. They rarely ask about the different levels of consultants to understand which level is the most capable for frontline consulting with the best value for dollars spent.

Potential clients also rarely ask how the consulting firm incentivizes its consultants. Not knowing can lead to mistrust. When only a few consultants are on-site every day, or all leave on a Thursday afternoon, are they reducing their costs to your project's disadvantage? When there are seemingly too many on-site, are they deliberately increasing your travel expenses? The answer to both questions is no, but without understanding how firms incentivize their consultants, it is easy to believe the worst and for trust to erode.

STRUCTURE AND CULTURE

Just as hospitals have organizational structures comprising managers, directors, vice presidents, and so forth, consulting firms have their own hierarchies. Titles differ across firms for the same roles (an analyst in one firm may be an associate in another). However, in general, the structure includes senior and junior levels of three categories: *associates, consultants,* and *directors* (exhibit 5.1).

Associates, or data analysts, are entry-level employees typically straight out of undergraduate programs. They may possess no consulting experience but are high achievers, great with data, and eager

Exhibit 5.1 Consulting Firm Structure

Managing Directors
Directors
Associate Directors
Senior Managing Consultants
Managing Consultants
Consultants
Senior Associates
Associates

to gain the experience and skills required to advance to senior associate and eventually consultant level. These young men and women work long hours to collect and pore over data, answer queries, prepare presentations, and take meeting minutes. They do whatever is necessary, glamorous or not, to provide the information that the senior consultants need to diagnose problems, make recommendations, and implement change.

Consultants, managing consultants, and senior managing consultants are the firm's subject matter experts. They are to consulting firms what doctors are to hospitals, teachers to schools, and lawyers to law firms. They provide the core service that clients pay for. You should be concerned if a consulting firm is deploying associates to perform the work of consultants. Doing so is cheaper for the firm but is like using medical students as doctors. As a hospital CEO, I once engaged a firm to help the physicians improve cost and quality. The firm sent an associate to the first meeting to present the cost and quality data findings. This was appropriate, and I had no concerns until the associate noted, to my surprise, that he was also functioning as a "change partner," a role he described as helping the physicians identify ways to improve their results. The latter function requires a consultant at least, and a good one to boot. I suspect the firm, trying to save costs, figured the associate had enough executive presence to pull it off. That was a mistake. It quickly became evident that the associate was out of his depth. This hurt the engagement and the credibility of the consulting firm.

Directors are the next category of consulting personnel. Each director typically leads a small consulting team, such as a revenue cycle team or labor team. Directors are the most experienced frontline personnel.

Managing director is the highest rung on the consulting team ladder, just below the leadership roles of the founders, CEO, and senior operational executives. Managing directors have two main roles. The first is to land engagements. In fact, sales ability is usually a prerequisite to becoming a managing director. The second role is to lead engagements. In this role, the managing director makes sure the whole engagement is progressing as planned and that the client's CEO and senior executives are happy. (As a managing director, I took action when the consultant "Jake" in chapter 4 was unable to implement his recommendations.) Managing directors also help directors and their teams interpret results and develop recommendations.

CASE 6

A large teaching hospital in California issued an RFP for a consulting firm to conduct a comprehensive performance improvement engagement. Several firms responded. After interviews, one emerged as the leading candidate. This firm was large and had the most resources and experience. It brought an impressive cast of managing directors and directors to the interview, and its sales deck featured several similarly sized academic medical center clients. Nevertheless, the hospital's evaluating team held some concerns. First, the firm was rigid in its methodology. The hospital leaders wanted to be involved in planning the engagement methodology and execution. They wanted to select the data analysis tools and have the hospital's faculty–researchers conduct data analysis. The consulting firm stated that strict adherence to its tried-and-tested methodology was necessary for success, and insisted on using its own data analysis tools and analysts.

The leading firm's price was also high, and instead of expressing a willingness to negotiate, the sales team asserted a "you get what you pay for" argument that the hospital interviewers perceived as arrogant. In addition,

→

the firm was not willing to put as much of its payment at risk as the hospital leaders desired. Finally, the most impressive sales team members admitted they only would be involved peripherally in the engagement.

Mindful of these concerns, the hospital leadership team decided to interview one more firm, "ABC Consulting," before making a decision. They had not planned to interview ABC because it was new, small, and relatively unknown in the industry. When invited to present, ABC brought fewer managing directors but more directors and senior managing consultants who would actually work on the engagement. Although the firm was new, the team noted proactively in its sales presentation that each of its consultants was highly experienced, having worked for many years at other consulting firms. Some had even worked at the leading firm. In contrast to the leading firm, ABC offered a high degree of flexibility in methodology. In addition, because it was highly motivated to land its first large client and had less corporate overhead than larger firms, ABC agreed to reduce its price and place more than the typical amount of its payment at risk. The hospital selected ABC Consulting, and the engagement was a success.

LESSONS

1 When hiring a consulting firm, qualifications and experience are essential but insufficient by themselves, just as when hiring an employee. The chemistry, or fit, with your culture also is critical, as is the consulting firm's motivation to meet your needs and support your mission. Beware when a consulting firm persists in trying to sell you what it has (such as particular programs, services, or cookie-cutter methodology) rather than what you need. It is easy to detect such firms: You leave the presentation feeling that they were not listening to you.

2 Ask who from the firm will work on your engagement and, in particular, who will lead the consulting teams. Do not assume that the best or most senior presenters will be the best on-the-ground consultants.

3 Set your engagement goals before you interview consulting firms. Expect firms to be flexible if they really want your business, and be wary when you encounter inflexibility. It may mean the firm has too many clients for its size and therefore does not have the bandwidth to be flexible, or worse, it may just have an arrogant culture.

Rather than requesting that all members of a sales team (which may be heavy in managing directors) work on your engagement, request a team with more of the hands-on experts such as consultants, managing consultants, senior managing consultants, and directors. This approach will also minimize your engagement price. Hourly rates vary from firm to firm, but managing directors commonly have billing rates of $450 to $800 per hour, in contrast to the consultant category of $250 to $450. Associates may cost $125 to $250. Every engagement needs managing directors, but having too many raises your price without delivering commensurate returns. Whether the firm charges a fixed fee or an hourly fee, the calculation usually involves multiplying the consultants' hours by their hourly rates.

KNOWING WHO'S THE BOSS

One nuance that distinguishes the hierarchy of hospitals from that of consulting firms pertains to the worker's functional boss. In hospitals, the leader above you is your boss. Consultants, however, spend most of their time at their clients' hospitals, not in their firm's offices. That is why the day-to-day hierarchy of a consulting firm is more functional: Whoever leads an engagement is the boss for that engagement, regardless of rank. If a director leads an engagement, all who work on that engagement—including managing directors—take instructions from that director. The ultimate functional boss, however, is always the client. For hospital employees, this would be analogous to the patient being in charge. For consultants, "the customer comes first" is not a lofty aspiration. It is real. This is good for you as the client. It means you have immense power over your consultants; you can ask them to redo work, and you can even micromanage the whole engagement, if that is your style.

Remember, though, that what you say carries weight. So if you express dissatisfaction with a consultant, the firm will likely remove that individual from the project, and sometimes from the consulting company. If you can temper your criticism by saying that a particular aspect of the consultant's performance is dissatisfying, then the engagement director will likely coach the offending consultant or change that consultant's duties for the project. Similarly, if you as the boss request a meeting for 5 p.m. Friday, consultants will fly in specifically for that meeting or delay their travel home for the weekend. This can make for an expensive meeting, and, from a work–life balance perspective, it can also hurt consultants' morale. If you give the consultants permission to call into the meeting, you will incur less expense and have happier consultants.

COMPENSATION AND INCENTIVES

Naturally, consultants' compensation and incentives depend on their rank. Senior experts such as managing directors have higher fixed salaries, but the firm will calculate their salaries based on the sales revenue it expects them to generate. The firm may lower managing directors' salaries if they miss sales targets. Managing directors and directors also typically participate in a bonus pool that fluctuates according to how much the year-end gross margin of the practice and firm exceeds a target. Although lower-level personnel such as associates and consultants earn less, their salaries usually are not subject to reduction because of missed sales targets. In addition, the firm typically guarantees some bonus based on individual performance, paying this bonus regardless of whether the firm meets its financial targets. The compensation and incentive structure for managing directors motivates them to (1) land engagements and sell services; (2) successfully complete the engagements, which leads to good references, which leads to more sales; and (3) achieve a preset gross margin on those engagements. As you can see, managing directors are highly incentivized to sell and to achieve targeted margins on those sales. You can use this motivation to your advantage in negotiations by offering the potential of additional engagements in the future or glowing references in return for a price discount.

Consulting firms' motivation to hit a preset gross margin for engagements is an important driver of their behavior. In fixed-fee engagements, the consulting firm wants to complete the engagement efficiently. The fewer consulting-hours expended to complete the project, the higher the margin. Problems arise when a consulting engagement drags on because of, say, a delay in scheduling meetings or resistance from the client's employees or physicians. If this continues, the consulting firm may exceed its internal budget for the engagement and its targeted gross margin will erode. In response, the firm may cut back on the number of consultants or the time each consultant spends on the engagement. This, in turn, will further delay the project, potentially leading to a failed project—a disastrous scenario for consulting firm and client alike.

You can prevent delays and avoid obstacles by designating an executive responsible for the engagement from the hospital's side. This leader not only holds the consultants accountable for meeting their deadlines and goals, but also holds your organization's employees and leaders accountable for helping the consulting firm succeed.

To achieve their targeted gross margin, consulting firms work hard to utilize their consultants as efficiently as possible across different client engagements. For example, if the consulting firm's internal budget for your engagement designates a revenue cycle consultant to spend two days a week on your site, the firm may schedule the consultant to spend the remaining two to three days at other client sites. This is not necessarily bad for you the client, because it ensures the consulting firm does not charge you for unnecessary consultant time. If, however, your engagement becomes inefficient, these external commitments can threaten the engagement's success. For example, if the consulting firm schedules your revenue cycle consultant to conduct interviews at your organization during the first week of the month and interviews at a different client's site during the second week, anything that prevents your meetings occurring during the first week could delay your interviews by at least two weeks. The more efficient you make the engagement, the better for both you and the consulting firm.

The firm's quest for good utilization also contributes to its drive for sales. Firms are motivated to minimize the amount of time consultants are "on the beach," that is, paid to sit at home after one engagement ends to when the next starts. If you are a firm's only client, the firm may be tempted to deploy more consulting hours on your engagement than needed. This is particularly true for time-and-materials contracts as discussed in the next chapter, "Setting the Price." This is one reason, as I also discuss in the next chapter, to set a not-to-exceed price.

ENGAGEMENT CHECKLIST

▶ **Have you appointed an executive responsible for leading the engagement on a day-to-day basis?**

This person will work with the consulting firm's engagement leader to ensure the engagement runs smoothly and efficiently. Choose someone with good project management, financial, data analysis, and interpersonal skills.

▶ **Do you have at least a general understanding of how the consulting firm incentivizes the consultants who work on your project?**

Given the proprietary nature of this information, not all firms will share it in the sales presentations, but most will be happy to share it in private.

▶ **How many other clients will your on-the-ground consultants be serving?**

It is normal for a firm to work with multiple clients simultaneously. If, however, the firm plans to spread your consultants across multiple engagements and some of the other clients are located far away, you should be concerned. Have a discussion with the firm about guaranteeing an adequate presence on your site. If the responses are not convincing, consider another firm.

CHAPTER 6

Setting the Price

> **CONSULTANT'S TIP**
>
> Be open to the idea of change. When clients aren't open to change, it's difficult for them to see the big picture or end goal. If those leaders and employees who resist consulting engagements focused more on collaboration with their consulting counterparts than on fighting them, they would realize that both parties have the same end goal: Both want to do what's best for the organization and patient experience.
>
> —*Senior associate, labor consulting*

BECAUSE CONSULTING FIRMS are highly motivated to win your project, you have the power to negotiate a good price. The challenge is estimating what that price should be, because there is no standard price for, say, conducting a three-month assessment. The absence of standard prices is in part because hospitals differ in size, and in part because engagements vary widely in scope and degree of difficulty.

To determine the right price, it is helpful to understand how consulting firms approach their internal budgeting for engagements. They start with cost inputs. The main drivers of the consulting firm's cost, and therefore your price, are the mix, utilization, and hourly rates of consultants. In accordance with the scope of your project, firms will estimate the composition and utilization of the consulting team—that is, how many associates, consultants, and other levels of experts they will deploy, for how many months, and the number of hours per week each team member will work on the project. The firm then simply multiplies each consultant's total hours by an hourly rate that incorporates indirect and other costs as well as the firm's preset margin. The firm may add the cost of tools such as software for revenue-cycle projections to this amount. The resulting price is not necessarily the price that the consulting firm quotes. Firms worry about underestimating the hours, size of the consulting team, or duration of the project, which would eat into their margins. For that reason, they may include a contingency amount, such as additional consulting hours that they might not eventually use.

Firms also worry about pricing themselves out of a sale, so they avoid boosting the price beyond the client's comfort zone. That explains the first rule of negotiation with consulting firms: Never answer their question, "What is your budget for this engagement?" If you do, your budget may become the consulting firm's price, even if the firm could have accomplished the engagement for less.

Some firms may not build in any cushion. Instead, they will quote their best estimate but with the caveat that you will pay for time and materials. This means that you cover all the hours and tools the firm provides regardless of whether the engagement is efficient or the firm hits its promised financial targets. Under a time-and-materials model, the consulting firm bears no risk. You will pay more than the estimated price if the engagement duration exceeds initial projections. The one advantage of this model for you is that it ameliorates the fear among employees and physicians that consultants in a risk-based payment model will lay off employees unnecessarily or disregard quality to hit a financial target.

If you accept a time-and-materials payment model, mitigate the downside by setting a not-to-exceed amount for the whole engagement. This incentivizes the consultants to work efficiently and quickly. Another common approach is to make at least some small portion, say 10 to 20 percent, of the consultant's payment at risk.

You pay the firm the at-risk portion only if the engagement achieves its financial targets, and you pay the rest as time and materials.

NEGOTIATING LEVERS

During negotiations, consulting firms can reduce their prices in six main ways, which are your potential negotiating levers. These are:

1. Decreasing or eliminating any cushion
2. Decreasing the proportion of expensive senior consultants
3. Decreasing the overall number of consultants
4. Decreasing the estimated number of hours per consultant
5. Decreasing the estimated length of the project
6. Decreasing the hourly rates

Of course, another way is to decrease the scope of the engagement, but this can reduce the engagement's benefit.

Before you start squeezing the consulting firm, however, remember that it is fair to pay a reasonably estimated price. If you pare margins excessively, you may cause the firm to skimp on necessary personnel or give your project low priority. The words "reasonably estimated" are important here, because not every consulting firm initially builds what the client might consider a reasonable internal budget. A large firm with slow sales and too many underutilized consultants may allocate more consultants to your project than you need. This will unnecessarily elevate the price.

To negotiate effectively, it is probably clear by now that you must understand the consulting firm's internal budget. It is standard for firms to provide this detail, including the number and mix of consultants they plan to deploy, for how long, and at what hourly rates. If they do not, ask for this information; if possible, ask before the firm quotes a price. This prevents the firm from backing into the number, mix, and hourly rate of the consultants to justify a price it already quoted.

SAVINGS GENERATORS

After you gather the internal budget details and initial price quote, a few negotiating approaches are open to you. Each of these tactics can successively generate more savings:

1. Accept the firm's quoted price if it appears reasonable.
2. Negotiate the price to a reasonable level, and then accept this price. This usually entails pushing back on the mix or number of consultants, the number of hours, or the hourly rates. Consider, for example, that an engagement's data collection phase requires fewer consultants than subsequent phases.
3. Negotiate the price to a reasonable level, and then ask the firm to reduce its price even more. This degree of price reduction usually requires you to reduce the scope of the engagement or reduce the engagement duration. You can also simply ask the firm to accept the lower price for the same scope and duration. In effect, you are asking the firm to accept lower margins. As mentioned earlier, firms might accept lower margins if they believe the current engagement could lead to more sales.

CASE 7

A 250-bed hospital in Texas selected a consulting firm to perform a comprehensive performance improvement engagement. The firm quoted a time-and-materials price of $3 million, which included 12 months of implementation consulting in the areas of labor, nonlabor/ supply chain, revenue cycle, and clinical performance improvement, yielding a projected $10 million in financial

→

CASE 7
(continued)

improvement. The firm based its price on a mix of consultants and associates working 176 hours per month (44 hours per week), at an average, or blended, rate of $200 per hour. It also included a senior consultant (managing director) serving as client services director, at a rate of $250 per hour for 20 hours per week, and software tools for approximately $100,000. The firm requested a time-and-materials contract rather than a risk-based contract. Although the firm believed the financial target was achievable, the consultants worried that the client's installation of a systemwide electronic health record at the same time could negatively affect their ability to achieve the financial target.

The hospital CEO and chief financial officer (CFO) countered with a price of $2 million with the following changes to the model:

1. Reduction in the client services director's on-site presence to 1½ days per week, 8 hours per day, for a total of 12 hours per week rather than the quoted 20 hours. The CEO and CFO successfully argued that client services directors, whose role is to manage the relationship with the client, did not need so many hours on-site to be effective. In most smoothly running engagements, a visit to the client site every other week is sufficient.

2. Reduction in the other consultants' on-site presence to four 8-hour days per week, for a total of 32 hours per week rather than the quoted 44 hours per week. The rationale was that consultants typically travel to a client's site on Monday morning and leave Friday mid-day, or even Thursday evening— they do not

CASE 7
(continued)

generally work five days a week. For purposes of pricing, it is also standard practice to consider a consultant's on-site workday as eight hours.

3. Further reduction in the cost of the project to ensure a 5:1 return. The hospital leaders proposed paying the consulting firm $2 million for a $10 million return. Their rationale, drawn from their experience, was that a 5:1 or greater return was reasonable; a 3:1 return was not.

In addition, the CEO and CFO required that the consulting firm put $700,000 of its payment at risk for achieving the target. They also set a $2 million not-to-exceed amount to ensure that any delays in the engagement, or cost overruns, would not lead to an increase in the total price. With minor changes, the consulting firm agreed to the counterproposal.

LESSONS

1 Always negotiate. Remember the consulting firm really wants your business and will typically price the engagement with some flexibility in mind.

2 Understand how the consulting firm built its initial price, and then push back on cost drivers that appear unrealistic or unnecessary. It is unrealistic to assume that consultants would fly to an engagement on Sundays and leave on Friday nights for the duration of the engagement, and it is unnecessary for a client services director to be spending 2½ days on-site every week. It follows that to negotiate effectively, you must understand the roles of the different consultants working on your engagement.

3 Even if you cannot guide the firm on how exactly to reduce the price, ask it to reduce the price to a point at which your return on investment (ROI) makes sense. The firm will know how to do this. It might reduce the number or mix of consultants or even the quoted hourly rate.

4 Try to place some of the payment at risk. Otherwise, the consulting firm has less incentive to run an efficient project and to hit the target.

5 Cap your payments at a certain not-to-exceed number. Consulting firms like to up-sell to increase revenues. Without a cap on the price, your final payments may exceed your initial price.

The negotiation option in which you negotiate the price to a reasonable point and then accept it best achieves the balance of cutting your price meaningfully but not so deep that the consulting firm performs a shoddy engagement. The negotiation option of asking the firm to discount even further becomes your logical approach if you still cannot afford the reasonable price. If at this point you still are not comfortable with a steeply discounted price, reconsider whether you truly have the funding for a consulting engagement. Even at the negotiation stage, it is not too late to back out. In fact, the specter of losing the engagement may cause the consulting firm to identify savings or funding approaches that you had not contemplated.

One way to pay as little from your existing funds as possible is to negotiate an agreement in which the consulting firm puts a large proportion of its payment at risk. In effect, you pay with dollars the consulting firm generates. Caution is necessary here. Every organization loves the idea of paying the consulting firm only after the organization "gets paid," but this type of financing is not always as great as it sounds. Consulting firms still will demand that some of their payment be fixed (not at risk), and in large engagements, this can be substantial. Firms also will not put their travel expenses at risk. Again, this payment can mount up, especially in large engagements. In addition, many firms will stipulate that your ROI under an at-risk model be less than that for a fixed-fee model, so what was a nice 5:1 return may now become a less-exciting 3:1 return. Finally, even if an at-risk deal looks great, you should realize that "getting paid" does not necessarily mean you will have the cash to pay the consulting firm. This is because when you pay a consulting firm, you do so in real dollars, whereas when a consulting firm computes what it has generated for you, it does so partly in real dollars and partly in so-called financial "opportunities." These opportunities are either initiatives that the firm has identified but you must implement after the firm leaves, or initiatives that the firm has implemented but will yield financial improvement incrementally over several months. In both cases, you will not see a portion of the financial improvement until after the engagement has ended, and getting paid, or at least getting fully paid, relies in part on the ability of your team to either implement or sustain initiatives.

CONSULTANT'S TIP

Take ownership and believe in the change.

—*Associate director, nonlabor/supply chain consulting*

ENGAGEMENT CHECKLIST

▶ Do you understand how the consulting firm arrived at its price?

Ask the firm for its budgeting methodology. Understandably, the firm will not share proprietary information, such as its targeted gross margin for the engagement, or information that could hurt the firm's negotiating position, such as how much contingency it has built into the price. However, it will share other vital information such as the mix, utilization, duration on-site, and hourly rates of the consultants. Hold a meeting with the leader from the consulting firm and your organization's CFO to understand the firm's assumptions. Then push back on any possibly excessive costs such as hourly rates or resources that are too rich for a given phase.

▶ Have you considered placing some of the firm's payment at risk and capping payments?

Be wary about accepting a time-and-materials price. When the consulting firm bears no financial risk for delivering on its projections, theoretically there is no limit to your payments. If the engagement becomes prolonged or the scope creeps, you still have to pay. A better approach is to place some payments at risk and the rest fixed rather than for time and materials. If you do accept a time-and-materials price, establish a not-to-exceed amount.

CHAPTER 7

Controlling Travel Expenses

CONSULTANT'S TIP

To resolve issues, clients should embrace us as partners in the process. We, as consultants, need to create an environment that allows open and honest dialogue. Projects work much better when clients and consulting teams seek the right answers together because successful partnerships yield the most significant results.

—*Managing director, integrated data management consultant*

AFTER YOU NEGOTIATE the engagement price, you must agree on the consulting firm's travel expenses for hotels, airfares, meals, and so forth. Consulting firms bill their travel expenses to clients as a "pass through." In other words, they do not include any markup and therefore have no incentive to inflate travel costs. They want to avoid shouldering any travel expenses and having a travel budget so limited that it interferes with project logistics or hurts their consultants' morale. Your goal, on the other hand, is to ensure that the consulting firm takes responsibility for keeping travel expenses as low as possible. Start by setting a cap, or not-to-exceed amount. Unless you set the cap too high, it will prompt the consulting firm to self-police expenses. Most firms will suggest a cap on travel expenses because they know clients expect it.

However, a cap shifts the risk from client to firm, so some firms will try to avoid it.

The cap is usually a percentage of the total price of the project. For example, setting travel expenses at 18 percent for a $1 million engagement means that you will cover travel expenses of up to $180,000 in addition to the $1 million fee. The percentage matters. Too high and, particularly for large engagements, your responsibility can be substantial; too low and the consulting firm will reach the cap before the engagement is complete. Regardless of the cap, consulting firms will never pay for travel out of their own pockets. This is understandable. To them, that would be like paying the hospital for the privilege of doing work for the hospital. That is why the consulting firm will ask for an increase when it approaches the cap. If you decline, the firm will reduce the amount of travel and, consequently, reduce the effort on your project. Thus, it is in your interest to be fair. A fair range for caps is 15–18 percent, but you could set the cap even lower, say 13 percent, with an agreement that you will increase it if necessary. Even the thought of a "we are approaching the cap" discussion with a hospital's chief financial officer (CFO) serves as motivation for most consulting firms to closely monitor and limit their expenses. At the same time, your commitment to elevating the cap if necessary assures the firm that you understand its position, and in light of the low initial cap, you will be reasonable.

Still, even consulting firms that are effective at self-policing their travel expenses can practice greater vigilance. Some consultants book hotels and airplane tickets late and consequently pay

---

CONSULTANT'S TIP

To drive revenue enhancement and cost reduction, clients must commit to the process and be ready to make difficult decisions. Executives need to own the engagement and model the behavior they want to see in their management and staff.

—*Managing consultant, labor*

---

unnecessarily high rates. Others charge for inappropriate items such as in-flight Internet service so they can work on multiple projects while traveling. In one egregious reimbursement request I reviewed, a consultant submitted a receipt for chewing gum that he bought in the airport.

Firms can only monitor their consultants' travel expenses after the fact, because receipts are turned in and reviewed at month's end. At that point, the firms have two options: pass the expense onto the client or eat the cost. They are loath to do the latter. Although reputable firms will never pass inappropriate expenses onto the client (the chewing gum charge never made it to the client), they also will not eat the costs of excesses such as late-booked hotel rooms and airplane tickets—travel is hard, and consultants will quit if they have to pay any part of it.

The retroactive nature of travel expense reimbursement makes it important that you ask the consulting firm to submit invoices in a timely fashion. That way, you can identify and curb troubling charges and trends early. I have seen situations where busy consultants have submitted travel expenses months after the expense occurred. This is too late to make any corrections. When consultants are overly tardy, predicting whether travel expenses will breach the cap and by how much can be impossible.

CASE 8 In 2011, a hospital in Washington State hired consultants to perform a comprehensive performance improvement engagement. The hospital and the consulting firm negotiated a travel expense cap of 15 percent of the total engagement fee. In addition, the hospital required the consulting firm to follow a detailed and rigorous travel expense policy created specifically for the engagement.

→

The policy included the following stipulations:

Rental cars: The cap on rental cars is $40 per day, with the requirement that consultants decline the prepay gas option and GPS units. Consultants should carpool when arriving at the airport on the same day.

Hotel: Maximum reimbursable hotel rate is set at $80 plus taxes. Consultants should use the hospital hotel for patients' families whenever rooms are available.

Food: The per diem rate for food is $37.50. Consultants should eat in the hospital cafeteria. Also, alcohol is not reimbursed.

Airfares: No first-class travel and no airfares above $800 are allowed without prior approval. Except in unavoidable situations, consultants must book all flights at least two weeks in advance.

This travel expense policy kept expenses lower than typical in engagements and below the 15 percent cap. The inconvenience of subpar hotels and the rental car and flight restrictions prompted some consultants to avoid traveling to that hospital and staying for prolonged periods. Fortunately, this reaction did not affect the overall engagement, which was successful.

LESSONS

1 This hospital was smart to implement a travel expense policy for its consultants. Without a policy, consultants can rack up large bills that include alcohol, expensive hotels, and inefficiently booked air tickets and rental cars.

2 Conversely, an onerous travel expense policy will lead consultants to travel less to your location than to other clients. This is particularly true with senior consultants, such as managing directors, who determine their own travel schedules and frequently work on multiple engagements. Consultants have harsh travel schedules. A nice hotel, good meals, and convenient logistics can make all the difference in their commitment to an engagement. Try to strike a balance between keeping the consultants happy and keeping travel expenses low.

3 In this case, the client created a new policy tailored to the engagement. A simpler and quicker approach is to modify the travel expense policy that already exists for your employees.

Rather than merely preventing the consulting firm from breaching the travel-expense cap, your negotiating goal should be to pay the least amount of travel expenses possible without hurting the engagement. Start this vigilance during the interview process by giving preference to qualified firms whose travel costs are inherently efficient because of their proximity to your hospital. In addition, during the engagement, request phone or video conference meetings when the consultants' in-person presence is not essential—there are many such meetings. To minimize travel expenses further, rent apartments for consultants rather than book pricey hotel rooms.

Always be clear that you will not pay for time spent traveling to your location. A consultant should not charge you for time spent sitting in an airport or plane. If the consulting firm has a client near your site, agree to pay only your prorated share of travel expenses.

Some might argue that clients do not need to take additional actions to constrain travel expenses. Most consulting firms already have a travel policy. As noted earlier, they gain nothing from exceeding the travel expense cap and dread conversations with CFOs questioning travel expense overruns. If you do not want to micromanage travel expenses and prefer instead to adopt the consulting firm's travel policy, first be sure that it is at least as rigorous as your organization's policy. Still, some degree of micromanagement is prudent. Although consulting firms do not benefit financially from travel expenses, they avoid placing too many restrictions on their consultants, so you can usually find some trims to make.

Finally, remember to strike a balance when setting travel rules. Good consulting firms will agree to reasonable expense restrictions, but it is important not to be so frugal that you lose valuable goodwill and damage your engagement.

CONSULTANT'S TIP

The leadership team should communicate to staff and physicians why the consultants were engaged, what the goals and scope of the consultation are, and how the engagement's timeline will proceed. The communication should emphasize that the engagement is a system initiative rather than a consulting firm initiative.

—*Senior managing consultant, perioperative*

ENGAGEMENT CHECKLIST

▶ **Have you set a travel expense cap?**

Do not necessarily accept the cap that the consulting firm initially quotes. If it is too high for your budget, counter with your own.

▶ **Have you determined and communicated a travel expense policy?**

Once you have set a cap, ask the consulting firm to explain its travel policy. Compare it to your organization's policy. Either accept the firm's policy, create a new one, or adapt the policy you use for employees. Whichever route you take, ask your finance department to track expenses and monitor adherence to the policy.

▶ Is someone in your purchasing office reviewing the firm's travel expenses?

It might not be cost-effective to review each item the consulting firm submits for reimbursement, but someone in your organization should review all large items such as airfares and hotel bills and periodically sample smaller items. Most consulting firms have a travel-expense software program, so ask for customized reports to make your job easier.

▶ Does the consulting firm have other clients in your vicinity?

If this is the case, or becomes the case during your engagement, be sure you are only paying your share of travel expenses.

CHAPTER 8

Communicating the Engagement

CONSULTANT'S TIP

The need for broad and continued communication from all levels of management holds true for both the success of the project as well as the project's impact on the care of patients. While the executive team is involved in most aspects of a project, managers and directors may not grasp the details of why changes are being made. Patient care is a continuous process of handoffs. When those processes change, communication is critical.

—*Director, labor consulting*

KEYS TO A GOOD START

Hospital employees and physicians frequently harbor negative feelings about consultants. They might believe consulting engagements portend a loss of jobs or represent a waste of money. Perhaps the organization is consultant fatigued, having gone through several engagements in recent years. Such fatigue is almost certain when the engagements are unsuccessful. How you communicate the decision to hire consultants is crucial to the overall success of the engagement. If you fail to assuage employees' fear and cynicism, the engagement will be suboptimal or fail completely.

Good communication of a consulting engagement starts before communication of the engagement itself. It begins with an explanation of the problem—the "burning platform"—that is forcing you to take a fateful leap (Conner 2012). Employees who do not know that their organization is financially distressed are unprepared to accept the need for a consulting firm. Although leaders might reveal that distress to employees, some avoid stating the true depth of the problem or the dire prognosis absent intervention. They may feel embarrassed, helpless, or worried about their own job security. In other cases, the leaders are like gamblers who think they can solve the mounting problem on their own before others become aware. Regardless, it is always self-defeating to bring in consultants without having first communicated the problem to the organization.

Communicating the urgency of a burning platform answers a fundamental employee question: "Why does the organization need to do anything different?" Once you have answered this question, another question may follow: "Why have you chosen to bring in expensive consultants rather than solving the problem internally?" (Actually, the first question in employees' minds is always, "Am I about to lose my job?" I will come back to that later.) If you have read chapter 2, you know how to answer the "why can't we fix things internally?" question because you had to answer it for yourself (see exhibit 2.1). The answer always includes the bandwidth or expertise, or a combination of both, to solve the problem in a timely manner.

You have a couple of concerns to address proactively: "What will the relationship be between me and the consultants? Do they answer to me? Do I answer to them?" The correct response is to explain that the consulting firm will be an extension of the leadership team and employees—"they will be us." This point is crucial. At all costs, avoid the us-versus-them mentality. That mindset has doomed many engagements. Success depends on the employees trusting, valuing, and even liking the consultants. How you launch, communicate, and manage the engagement enforces the "they will be us" message. By the way, favor consulting firms that mirror that message with the assurance that "we will be you."

| **CASE 9** | A 350-bed faith-based hospital in California hired a consulting firm to conduct a comprehensive performance improvement engagement. |

The hospital CEO called a meeting with physicians, where he explained that his key reason for hiring the consultants was to reduce the "unacceptable costs of care." He strongly urged the physicians to work with the consultants, adding that the consultants would receive one of every five dollars generated in financial improvement. At this revelation, the perturbed physicians began furiously texting each other. The meeting quickly devolved into physicians questioning the wisdom of hiring expensive consultants, blaming administration for the hospital's strategic missteps, and demanding data to support the contention that the hospital's costs of care were excessive. Following the meeting, many of the physicians shunned the consulting engagement. The results of the engagement were suboptimal.

LESSONS

1 Leaders must not appear to blame incumbents when introducing consultants to an organization. It is counterproductive for employees or physicians to view your decision to hire consultants as a criticism of them. Here, the physicians interpreted the "unacceptable costs of care" rationale as code for "physicians are to blame." A better approach would have been for the CEO to say, "I have informed the consultants about the great work you do each day, and I have asked them to help us become more affordable for patients." Blame creates resentment, suspicion, and opposition.

2 Transparency is important, but be careful how you communicate details of consultants' compensation, particularly before the consultants have a chance to demonstrate value. Until physicians and employees see promised financial and operational improvements from the engagement, they will believe that the consultants are overpaid. It is particularly unwise for a leader to communicate to physicians and employees that the hospital will pay the consultants solely according to financial targets. Such incentives will make the physicians fear the consultants might sacrifice quality for earnings and will make employees fear for their jobs. A wiser approach is to create incentives that also include maintaining or improving quality of care.

Speaking Honestly

Let's consider the first question on each employee's mind: "Is my job in jeopardy?" Carefully think through your answer even before you hire the consultants. If the honest answer is "maybe," then how you communicate it will be crucial to avoid widespread panic and resistance. The best response is to say the consultants will look at all opportunities for improvement, and it is too early to tell whether this will involve staffing changes. You should also commit to keeping employees informed as the evaluation progresses. Admittedly, this message is not what employees want to hear, but it is honest and logical. If you know the consultants will not recommend layoffs (i.e., you have instructed the firm that staffing reductions should occur only by attrition and not filling vacancies), then state that early and emphatically. Employees will breathe a collective sigh of relief, and then most subsequent discussions will go smoothly.

The message is much trickier if you engaged the consultants specifically to reduce your organization's headcount. Even here, honesty is still the best policy. Start by avoiding eye-rolling terms such as *rightsize*, and instead be direct, genuine, and empathetic. Tell the employees that because of the burning platform problem, you must reduce staffing costs. Explain that you hired the consultants to help you gain a better understanding of the organization's current work and future needs, so that you and the organization—not the consultants—can make thoughtful decisions that protect the mission and treat employees fairly. Describe how difficult these decisions will be for you personally, and express a commitment to supporting affected employees in their transitions. There is no way to make employees like this message, but if you express it thoughtfully, many will respect your honesty, understand the necessity to reduce staffing, and view interaction with the consultants as an opportunity to demonstrate their value.

Still, the specter of layoffs hurts employee morale, and when morale suffers, an organization's operations may feel negative effects. To avoid this consequence, some hospitals only use attrition, not layoffs, to reduce staffing costs. Of course, employees must understand

---

CONSULTANT'S TIP

Clients should fulfill data requests during the assessment phase as rapidly and completely as possible to allow for a thorough, complete, and accurate review. Clients should also be as open and transparent to ensure there are no blind spots. Then, leadership should not only communicate the intent of the engagement but also hold staff accountable for collaboration and follow-through. Clients who embrace a team approach, with us immersed in their culture, are more likely to see success.

—*Senior managing consultant, human resources*

that a "no layoffs" plan does not change the customary policy of reducing positions here and there according to the organization's needs. Employees will accept the attrition approach, and most consulting firms will be relieved because it allows them to start on the right footing with the employees. Consider adopting this approach. The result is frequently an amazing partnership between the consultant and client that drives a degree of financial and operational improvement well beyond their original expectations.

Building the Campaign

It is important that you communicate the consulting engagement to *all* employees. Failure to communicate widely leads to a common situation in which some employees are unaware of the engagement until the consultants arrive. This is an ominous way to start. Avoid this mistake by conducting a communications campaign that goes beyond existing channels such as employee forums, department meetings, and newsletters. Include personalized approaches such as a video message from the CEO and a dedicated consulting-engagement intranet site. You should not have to develop everything from scratch. Good consulting firms will have a toolbox of communication approaches and content gleaned from previous engagements.

This leads to the topic of naming, or branding, the engagement. Work with the consulting firm to develop an identity for the engagement. Avoid defaulting to the name of the consulting firm, because that would run counter to the idea that the consultants are an extension of the leadership team and employees. You do not want leaders and employees to view this as the consulting firm's project. You want them to view it as the organization's initiative. Even the word "project" or "engagement" in the name is unhelpful. It will make employees view it as just that—a short-term, narrow-scope endeavor, after which the hospital will return to business as usual. Furthermore, naming the engagement after the consulting firm is confusing because it really does not explain what the project is about.

The name you choose will depend on the type of engagement, but here are some examples:

- Cost and Value Campaign
- Clinical Efficiency and Effectiveness Assessment
- Clinical Sustainability Initiative
- Resource Utilization Management
- reCreate [name of hospital]

I am not suggesting that you adopt any of these names; each has pros and cons. The point is to create a compelling and descriptive name for your engagement before you launch your communications campaign.

Addressing Specific Audiences

During the communication campaign, some audiences merit special attention. These include physicians, labor unions, and perhaps performance excellence (PE) teams of Lean Six Sigma employees you use as internal consultants. These three stakeholder groups will resist consultants if not approached properly.

Why do I put PE teams on this list? Because PE teams may view the engagement of consultants as an act of no confidence in their work. In addition, PE teams are already conducting performance improvement efforts that they fear the consultants will usurp. You can mitigate resistance from PE teams by reassuring them that you value their efforts and will rely on their change management skills to help monitor and ensure the sustained success of the engagement. To prevent establishment of silos, allow your PE teams to report progress in their initiatives through the same engagement structure the consulting team uses to report its progress.

If your organization is unionized, you must meet early in the engagement with union leaders to explain your reasons for hiring a consulting firm and answer their questions. Their main interests will be to preserve their members' jobs and see that you do not breach any union agreement rules. If your answers worry them, they will oppose the engagement. A common union argument goes like this: "If your organization is in financial distress, why are you wasting money on high-priced consultants? Aren't you paid to handle this sort of problem?" Respond by describing the burning platform scenario to explain that the organization is in financial jeopardy; explain that your team lacks the bandwidth, expertise, or both, to address the enormity of the situation adequately. Also, tell them that you will employ an attrition approach to reducing staffing costs, if true. If staff reductions are likely, assure the union you will follow the terms of the collective bargaining agreement. Regardless of your communication efforts, the unions will take a wait-and-see view, at best. It is always important to give them frequent updates on the progress of the engagement, including specific initiatives you are implementing.

Your approach to addressing the medical staff is important, too. Most physicians will not understand why you need consultants, and many will criticize the cost of the engagement. If you ignore this skepticism, they might resist important initiatives such as flexible staffing of nurses and reduction of medical device costs. They might even resist the whole engagement. Recommendations on how to engage physicians could fill a whole book. In fact, I have written *An Insider's Guide to Physician Engagement* (Agwunobi 2018). With regard to consulting engagements, there are four important points for you to follow:

- *Communicate your burning platform.* Include the poor prognosis for both finances and possibly even patient care if you do not bring in help.
- *Provide them with valuable new data that can improve the physicians' work lives.*
- *Show them how the engagement can improve the operations of their clinics.*

- *Communicate that you will involve them in any decisions.* Include any issues that directly or indirectly affect physicians or patients.

CONSULTANT'S TIP

A communication plan should be developed and used throughout the consultation, including achievement of milestones.

—Senior managing consultant, perioperative

ENGAGEMENT CHECKLIST

▶ Have you communicated the burning platform to stakeholders?

Employees and other stakeholders are more likely to accept a consulting engagement if you have informed them the organization is in serious trouble. It is suboptimal practice to reveal the consulting engagement and the burning platform at the same time, but if you have not proactively communicated the problems beforehand, try to separate the topics because each needs its own focused discussion. First, communicate details of the burning platform and allow opportunities for questions and discussion. Then share the details regarding the consulting firm decision. This may require two meetings with all stakeholders.

▶ Have you prepared for the first question that will be on each employee's mind?

If you do not intend to lay off employees, then communicate this early and often. However, it is prudent to wait until you have discussed workforce changes with the consulting firm before making any guarantees. Some firms will welcome an attrition-based approach to staffing reductions; others will prefer to decide after completing the assessment. If you must wait to answer the question, at least express your desire not to reduce jobs. If you know layoffs will be necessary, be transparent but emphasize that the process will be rigorously vetted and fair. In addition, communicate that any affected employees will be supported and treated fairly.

▶ Have you prepared a robust communications campaign?

This is a plan that you should develop with your consultants because they will have tools and messages to help. Develop a customized plan for delivering content to your physicians—it is especially hard to get the attention of busy medical staff.

▶ Have you created a name for your consulting engagement?

The name should emphasize that the engagement is the organization's initiative. Involve the consulting firm and your senior executive team in the naming process. Some organizations involve all their employees to build excitement and involvement. Creating a name for your engagement should be one of the first tasks you undertake. The longer you wait, the more likely a default name, such as the (insert consulting firm name) project, will become misleading.

REFERENCES

Agwunobi, A. C. 2018. *An Insider's Guide to Physician Engagement.* Chicago: Health Administration Press.

Conner, D. 2012. "The Real Story of the Burning Platform." *Change Thinking* (blog). Posted August 16. www.connerpartners.com /frameworks-and-processes/the-real-story-of-the-burning -platform.

CHAPTER 9

Launching the Engagement

CONSULTANT'S TIP

The best results occur when a client is open to changing their processes to fit the new model, not by forcing old methods into new processes or new tools.

—*Director, labor consulting*

READY FOR LAUNCH

Now that you have prepared your employees for the engagement, you must actually launch it after addressing a couple of immediate needs.

Finding Space for the Consultants

This is usually an afterthought, and it is therefore usual for clients to give the consulting team crummy space such as an empty storage room or a mothballed set of patient rooms on an unused floor. Remember that consultants are essentially temporary employees. You want them to be engaged and productive, and you want them to become extensions of your leadership team and employees. You would not put a new vice president of operations in a trailer behind your loading dock. If the consultants' office space is inconvenient, uncomfortable, or far from the services they will evaluate and address, their performance and your results may suffer.

Frankly, how much the consultants like the space is important, too. Treat your consultants well and they will want to travel to your engagement and put in extra effort for superior results.

Integrating Consultants with Staff

To make consultants part of your organization's team, the effort must be real and intentional. Here, small things matter. For example, unless your organization is extremely formal, tell the consultants to dress down—business casual instead of the stereotypical corporate mafia look.

Don't overlook the big things, either. Make sure that a dyad comprising a consulting firm team leader and a leader from your organization leads each engagement workgroup. Furthermore, have the leaders from your organization (rather than the consultants) present the results of the workgroup so that your leaders begin to own the work. This will also motivate your leaders to understand the consultants' work and resolve any disagreements before the workgroup presents.

Another good way of avoiding an us-versus-them culture is to avoid holding any internal meetings about the engagement without the consultants present. Compelling your team to discuss any issues or concerns openly with the consultants prevents passive-aggressive resistance and unproductive criticism of the consultants. Open discussions also foster trust between the consultants and the executives and enable the consultants to address complaints immediately.

To emphasize a point made in chapter 8, "Communicating the Engagement," it is best to avoid calling the engagement by the name of the consulting firm. In fact, minimize the use of the firm's name or eliminate the word *consultants* altogether. Instead, refer to those working on the engagement/initiative as the *team* rather than the *consultants.* Give credit for accomplishments to the whole team—including your employees—not only the consultants.

Managing the Meetings

The launch starts with kickoff meetings where the consultants present to the various stakeholders, such as the board, senior executives, directors, managers, and physicians. These meetings allow the consulting team to introduce themselves and communicate their approach, the phases of the engagement, timelines, focus areas, and next steps.

These meetings are extensions of the communication campaign, and they are fraught with risks. You need to help the consultants deliver the right message and establish credibility with your organization. A wrong impression from the consultants can imperil the rest of the engagement. Keep a tight hold on the proceedings to ensure that the consultants' message aligns with yours. You want to see that their debut engenders confidence, their explanation of the project is clear, and that they avoid common consulting foibles such as making incorrect assumptions drawn from their experience with other clients.

The presentations of a firm that listens well may not require micromanagement. Still, the maxim "trust but verify" applies. Typically, you will modify some elements of their message, even if only minimally. Previewing their presentation slide decks will tell you whether change is necessary. The following are common problems.

- *Opening slides feel like a sales pitch.* Because sales are so important to consulting firms, and they sell so frequently, their introductory slides may come across as a sales pitch even after the firm has won the engagement. This misstep is a turnoff for internal stakeholder groups because it reinforces negative stereotypes of consultants as salespeople. I have even seen it confuse stakeholders into thinking they are interviewing the firm when the firm is actually launching the engagement. Help the consultants achieve a balance of impressing without slipping into the sales role. They can accomplish this by keeping the introductory slides brief and highlighting only a few impressive points about themselves such as the size of the firm, the number of similar engagements worked, and qualifications of key consultants.

- *The slides are generic.* During an engagement launch, some consulting firms will use the same slide deck for all the stakeholder groups. This is a mistake. Although it makes sense for some slides to be the same, the consultants should customize others for the audience. Physicians may be most interested in how the consultants plan to protect and enhance patient care, whereas senior executives may be most interested in how the firm will interact with department leaders or approach staffing reductions.

- *The slides are unclear.* You should expect sophisticated productions from consulting firms, and most deliver. However, some create slide decks that lack polish. I have seen slides that are cluttered, disjointed, unformatted, and titled with unclear headings. An unpolished slide deck does not necessarily mean the engagement will be bad, but it certainly conveys that impression to stakeholders. Give the consulting firm specific instructions on how to improve their slide deck for the audiences in your organization. They may be embarrassed, but they will appreciate your engagement and assistance in the end.

- *The slide deck is too long.* This is a nearly universal problem. Most consultants want to do more than merely give value for money; they want to give volume for money. This desire frequently translates into slide decks that can be a mind-numbing length of 50-plus slides. Tell your consultants to make their presentations as crisp as possible. One approach is for them to relegate all but the most necessary slides to an informational appendix.

- *The consultants haven't identified all the right stakeholder groups or are approaching them incorrectly.* Initially, consulting firms won't understand the dynamics of your organization. They might lump the wrong stakeholder groups together or completely miss important groups and individuals. For example, at one organization's engagement, the perioperative consultants planned to present to all the surgeons together. The client pointed out that the cardiac surgeons had their own dedicated (and sometimes competing) operating rooms, and it would be better to present to them separately. At other times, consultants may have the right stakeholder groups but not recognize the formal or informal leaders who, for courtesy or political reasons, must see a preview of the kickoff presentation. It is important to help the consultants understand all dynamics.

- *The presenters are bad.* During the sales presentation, it may become clear that one (or more) of the consultants is a poor presenter. They may come across as angry, denigrating, insensitive, or merely boring. I saw one presenter punctuate almost each statement with a long, noisy swig from a bottle of water. When there are bad presenters, privately ask the engagement director not to invite them to present at kickoff meetings. Unfortunately, you won't always have the opportunity to see how awful a presenter is until the kickoff meetings start, so it's a good idea to attend this meeting and provide extra assistance if needed. A more important reason to attend is to help the consultants gain acceptance by introducing them with a few supportive comments before they speak. Your comments should summarize your burning platform, list the reasons you selected these consultants, explain your confidence in them, and stress that they will be a great addition to the employees and leadership team.

| CASE 10 | A 150-bed hospital in Maryland engaged a consulting firm to conduct a financial and operational turnaround. In addition, the CEO asked the firm to provide an interim to fill the |

newly created position of chief transformation officer (CTO). Some executives resisted the idea of hiring the consultants, particularly a CTO from the consulting firm. The CEO, however, was determined to make the engagement a success. She directed that the interim CTO's office be located in the CEO's suite. She knew that placement would convey the importance and integrated nature of the interim CTO role. The CEO housed the remainder of the consultants in a conference room near the other senior executives, further emphasizing her message of importance and integration. She also wanted her executives to work closely with the consultants. The approach worked. Through daily interactions, the executives quickly came to view the consultants as an extension of themselves. The engagement became a shared endeavor that exceeded its financial targets.

LESSONS

1 Do not underestimate the symbolism and practical advantages of locating your consultants strategically. If you put them in a distant room or down in the basement, your employees and executives (when they remember the consultants even exist) will view them as peripheral to the mission.

2 Encourage organization leaders to accept and value the consultants, because employees will take their cues from leadership. Setting joint leader–consultant goals, such as a targeted increase in point-of-service cash collections for the chief financial officer and revenue cycle consultants, will motivate leaders to welcome the consultants' help and appreciate their expertise.

ENGAGEMENT ORGANIZATIONAL STRUCTURE

Prior to launching your engagement, create an engagement organizational structure of an executive steering committee (ESC) and workgroups. The main role of the ESC is to coordinate and monitor the engagement. It also allows you and your senior executives to guide the consultants, remove obstacles, and collect information to communicate to the rest of the organization. The workgroups coordinate the work of the specialized areas. For example, a labor workgroup would review labor data and staffing grids, support and coordinate staffing changes, and so on. In a comprehensive engagement, other workgroups might cover nonlabor/supply chain, revenue cycle, patient flow, human resources, perioperative, and clinical areas. There also could be subgroups for specific initiatives such as decreasing the use of expensive pharmaceuticals.

In a large engagement with many workgroups, meeting overload can occur. Too many time-consuming meetings will cause scheduling conflicts for employees, executives, and physician leaders and lead to poor attendance. Conversely, too few meetings can be counterproductive—for a four-month assessment, of course, monthly work group meetings are insufficient.

One way of finding the right balance is to piggyback engagement meetings onto existing organizational meetings and then keep the added portions brief. This approach works well for ESC meetings, which can be appended to weekly or biweekly senior executive team (SET) meetings. Specifically, consider allocating 20 minutes of the SET agenda for the ESC. Once a month, make the ESC portion longer—around 30–45 minutes—to enable deeper discussions.

During the ESC portions of the SET meetings, invite additional attendees as appropriate to the topics. You can apply this same piggybacking approach for workgroups. For example, instead of creating a new surgery workgroup, commandeer some time on the monthly operating room executive committee agenda.

In addition to ESC and workgroup meetings, hold executive sponsor meetings where you, as the sponsor, meet regularly with the consulting firm's engagement director. These meetings ensure that you will not be surprised with controversial information during the ESC. They also serve as safe forums where the engagement director can communicate information they prefer not to say in front of a broader audience. These sensitive topics might include resistance from members of the ESC, compliance-related discoveries, or political concerns such as how to handle queries from a board member.

CONSULTANT'S TIP

Share expectations early with stakeholders. Explain that a successful multimonth engagement requires cultural change and that results are not immediate.

—*Managing consultant, nursing*

ENGAGEMENT CHECKLIST

▶ **Have you selected a suitable location for the consultants' team room?**

If you are delegating this task to others, give them the criteria and make the final decision yourself. The space should be comfortable and include an office or two for the consultants to conduct interviews. If possible, locate the space close to administration or to the focal point of the engagement, such as the OR for a perioperative consulting engagement.

▶ **Have you worked with the consulting firm to create a manageable and effective engagement structure?**

This task includes creating dyads of consulting leaders and your executives to report progress at ESC meetings. It also includes working with the consultants to determine the number of workgroups and frequency of meetings. To conserve time, add brief engagement-related meetings onto existing meetings.

▶ **Have you reviewed the consulting firm's kickoff slide deck?**

Do not hesitate to review the consultants' deck. Most firms are used to this, and they should appreciate your guidance and engagement. Even if the presentation materials look great, your review will help the consultants align their overall message with your message.

Managing the Engagement

THE ASSESSMENT PHASE

Consulting engagements typically follow a simple model: an assessment phase followed sometimes by an implementation phase. During the assessment, the consultants collect and analyze your data, interview your employees, and observe workflows. The consultants then present their findings with a written report.

Dealing with Data Request Problems

Although the model is simple, several problems can complicate the process. These problems might even derail the assessment. Common problems and their solutions follow.

- *The shotgun data request.* At an assessment's onset, consulting firms make a formal data request for the information they need to understand your organization and identify areas for improvement. Data requests range from easy-to-supply information such as the organizational structure chart to complex financial, utilization, market share, and clinical outcomes. Gathering these data and confirming their accuracy can be difficult and time-consuming. The burden increases when consulting firms take a shotgun approach of asking for much more information than they need. Firms frequently argue that they need as much information as possible because "we don't know what we don't know." The truth is that firms typically will not review all the data they request. Their real reason for such broad requests is convenience. It is easier for firms to follow a standard data-request list they created years before and ask for everything than it is to recreate the request for each engagement.
- *Conflicting or inaccurate data.* Inaccuracies frequently result when firms send data requests directly to operational departments. The managers might misinterpret the requests, submit conflicting responses (particularly when requests go to multiple departments), or respond with erroneous data that the finance or other responsible department hasn't validated. For example, patient volume data from the cardiology department may differ from finance department data because finance will likely use claims data whereas cardiology will provide a log of visits. Also, when department managers are rushed, the data they send might be incomplete.
- *Privacy breaches.* Some of the data requested, such as organizational charts, may be public. However, protected health information and proprietary financial numbers are

confidential and must be shielded when your organization transmits that data to the consulting firm. Most consulting firms have secure file-sharing methods to receive and store information, but mistakes can occur. A common one occurs after a formal data request when a consultant asks a department manager for clarifying information, and the manager replies by sending the requested information by unencrypted e-mail.

To avoid these problems, set up a data planning team at the beginning of the engagement. At a minimum, this team must include the consulting firm's point person for issuing the data request and a counterpart at your organization who is responsible for your organization's responses. Because of the need for data validation and the amount of data the consulting firm typically requests, designating a person from finance is a good idea. The data planning team warrants that all requested data are necessary and eliminates duplicate requests. The team also ensures that data requests are clear in scope, the organization validates the data's accuracy, privacy is protected, and departments respond in a timely manner. No data requests should go to any department without first going through the data planning team.

CONSULTANT'S TIP

Clients should broadcast the goals of the engagement from the very top to the bottom of the organization and to vendors. They should make sure that the highest level of the organization supports the engagement. And they should help to drive the results throughout the organization, including physicians.

—*Managing consultant, nonlabor/supply chain*

Addressing Interview Problems

During the assessment phase, consultants conduct multiple interviews to supplement the data analysis. In a large engagement, interviews can exceed a hundred; they can involve board members, executives, department heads, physicians, and frontline employees. In such a large undertaking, several potential problems will merit your attention.

- *Unfocused interviews.* Lacking structure, interviews can make the engagement longer, costlier, and more disruptive than necessary. Issues arise when the consulting firm fails to customize its questions according to the findings from its data request. This becomes evident when the firm begins interviews before completing the data request phase. In unfocused interviews, generic questions predominate: "What do you think needs to improve?" or "How do you think the organization can save money?" The resulting superficial answers do not advance the engagement. For example, without analyzing the device or implant utilization of an orthopedic department, any interview of the orthopedic surgeons will likely yield low-value information. Conversely, focused interviews help consultants validate data findings and probe for solutions. With orthopedic surgeons, these data points could confirm the number of device vendors, identify physicians who are over-utilizers, and validate the levers for change.

  Unfocused interviews are problematic in other ways, too. Consultants inevitably interview stakeholders who don't need to be interviewed. Busy physicians, in particular, will find this vexing. And perhaps the largest downside of interviews conducted without the benefit of a foundational data analysis is that after the consultants complete the data analysis and identify opportunities for improvement, they will need to reinterview many individuals.

The most effective tactic is to make sure that the consulting firm schedules interviews to start after its data request. In addition, ask the consultants for examples of the questions they will be asking. Confirm that the consultants derived their questions from an understanding of the data.

- *Unprepared interviewees.* It is common for interviewees to be clueless about why they are meeting with the consulting firm. They arrive feeling anxious and guarded, and this feeling affects the quality of the interview. In addition, unprepared interviewees are unable to give sufficiently detailed answers. Often, consultants have no option but to ask them to think about the questions and then return later for a follow-up interview. This delays completion of the engagement. Direct the consulting firm to create an agenda and then send it in advance to interviewees. This should be more than a list of topics. It should begin with a few sentences explaining the engagement and the reason for the interviews. Review and edit this introductory language.

- *Overly lengthy interviews.* For some reason, many consulting firms feel that interviews have to be lengthy, sometimes as long as two hours. Most cite thoroughness as their rationale. Actually, lengthy interviews are more about the interviewers' habits. When the consultants ask focused questions and the interviewees are prepared, short interviews can be as productive as lengthy ones. One-hour meetings are sufficient for group interviews, and 30-minute meetings frequently work well for 1:1 interviews. Besides the gratitude of interviewees and limited disruption, shorter interviews yield a solid benefit for consultants: They will have time to conduct more interviews. To confirm that the consultants' interviews are reasonable, ask them to show you their interview calendar and then push back on interviews that are too long.

| CASE 11 | An academic hospital in Texas engaged a consulting firm to implement cost savings across the organization. The firm sent voluminous data requests to various |

department directors. Some requests were duplicative, and some departments didn't understand what the consultants were requesting. Citing concerns about efficiency, data accuracy, and privacy, the client halted the data request phase and worked with the consulting firm to improve the process. In the meantime, the consulting team launched and completed more than 60 interviews of executives and physician leaders. The executive interviews yielded useful insights, but many of the physician interviews did not. Some physicians arrived unsure about why they were meeting with consultants. Others had no idea why the hospital hired the consulting team, and a few were unaware of the fact that the hospital had hired consultants. To make matters worse, after the hospital and consultants relaunched the improved data request process and analyzed the responses, the consultants realized they would need to repeat many of the physician interviews to explore the information and opportunities the data revealed.

LESSONS

1 Do not let your consultants launch the interview process until after they have completed the data collection and analysis. A good analysis guides the interview questions and helps the consultants decide whom they should interview. Meeting with the chief of orthopedic surgery before knowing the number of device vendors and the associated costs is a wasted opportunity, and there is no reason to interview the chief of ob/gyn if no significant opportunities exist in that department.

2 Ensure that the consultants issue an agenda before each interview. Include a few sentences introducing the consultants and explaining the rationale for the engagement and the interviews.

Observing the Work

During the assessment phase, all consulting firms conduct data analyses and interviews, but some do not observe the work the employees perform. The complexity of hospitals makes thorough observation difficult, labor intensive, and costly, and a concern for costs is why some implementation firms will delay such observations until the beginning of the better-compensated implementation phase.

The problem with this delay is that clients are disappointed when they realize that, contrary to their assumptions, observations are not part of the assessment. Employees are unpleasantly surprised, and those who resist the engagement will point to the lack of observation as evidence of the invalidity of the consulting firm's recommendations. Therefore—before signing an agreement—make sure you understand how much workflow observation, if any, the consulting firm plans to conduct in the assessment. One way to mitigate costs is to have the consulting firm conduct targeted observations in only a few areas. Even a small amount of observation is helpful in both improving the consultants' understanding and preventing employee disappointment and resistance.

Vetting the Data

The credibility of an engagement suffers when consultants announce a great savings opportunity that you later find to be incorrect. In one case, for example, a consulting firm assessing a midsize hospital informed the CEO that the hospital could realize $900,000 in savings by improving the productivity of its hospitalist group. The CEO happily called for a meeting with his lead hospitalist and the consultants. But at this meeting, the CEO unhappily realized that the consultants had not only misunderstood the hospitalists' staffing model but also had applied outdated staffing benchmarks. The potential for $900,000 savings did not exist. In fact, citing the correct benchmarks, the lead hospitalist could have argued for more staff. This embarrassment occurred because the consultants had not vetted their information with the hospitalist group. That's why it is so important to require the consultants to vet all significant data before issuing recommendations.

Motivating Your Consultants

Essentially, consultants are temporary employees; like regular employees, they can become disengaged when they feel unsupported. The good news is that the same factors that motivate regular employees can work for consultants. The main motivator is positive feedback, which serves to validate their work. The more personal you make the validation, the more powerful the motivation will be. Consultants may feel underappreciated when clients treat them as invisible and emotionless invaders. Although you have no obligation to feel warm and fuzzy toward your hired guns, remember that the hired guns are actually hired humans, and humans have a basic desire to feel that they matter. In the final episode of *The Oprah Winfrey Show*, the host said, "I've talked to nearly 30,000 people on this show, and all 30,000 had one thing in common: They all wanted validation. . . . [E]very single person you will ever meet shares that common desire. They want to know: Do you see me? Do you hear me? Does what I say mean anything to you?" (Oprah.com 2011)

This feeling is true with consultants, particularly those new to the business. Whereas seasoned consultants might be hardened to a lack of validation and disrespect, new consultants haven't developed this protective shell. This treatment is especially painful for consultants who enter the field later in their careers from jobs in industry (such as a director of purchasing who becomes a supply chain consultant) because they are accustomed to positive feedback.

A few months after becoming a consultant, following many years as a hospital CEO, I and another senior consultant began a comprehensive performance improvement project for a large academic medical center in California. A few weeks into the engagement, a hospital director, who had been present when we introduced ourselves during the kickoff meeting, asked to meet with us. I thought he wanted to give pointers on opportunities. Instead, he started the meeting by saying, "I want to explain to you how academic hospitals work so that you can be most effective as consultants." The rest of the meeting was the equivalent of new employee orientation. Perhaps he was trying to help, but he either forgot or chose to ignore the fact that I had managed a large academic medical center and other hospitals for more than 12 years and that my colleague was a 17-year veteran of hospital performance improvement consulting. The director's assumption seemed to be that we could not possibly know much about the actual work of academic hospitals. I was demoralized, while my hardened colleague laughed it off. Maybe I was being overly sensitive. If so, that only underscores the vulnerability of new consultants and their need for validation. For most consultants, the monetary rewards, the esprit de corps of the team, and the occasional pat on the back from the team leader all motivate, but they don't fully substitute for the client's assurance that "you are doing good work, and your opinions matter."

Another way that clients inadvertently communicate disregard for their consultants is by scheduling meetings and then canceling them at the last minute for minor reasons. This is particularly disheartening to consultants after they have traveled a long distance to attend.

The main takeaway in this discussion (and a recurring theme in this insider's guide) is that you will get more from your consultants if you treat them with the same consideration as you treat your employees. You can accomplish this easily. Make it a habit to know the names and backgrounds of your consultants. Take the time to visit the consultants' team room or have lunch with them in the cafeteria. Give positive feedback, including writing thank-you notes or e-mails when consultants perform well. Be considerate of their time and difficult travel schedules.

Monitoring Progress

Chapter 12 addresses monitoring in detail and focuses on implementation rather than assessment phases because assessments are sometimes extremely short. Nevertheless, it is prudent at this point to highlight the need to monitor assessments, particularly if they are longer than two months. Without some monitoring, the assessment may be over and the invoice in your inbox before you realize the engagement has gone off the rails. Some unmonitored consultants may perform superficial assessments to constrain their costs and enhance margins. Avoid these problems by setting and monitoring milestones, and then require the consultants to report periodically on their progress toward identifying opportunities.

Reviewing the Recommendations

Following data collection, interviews, and observations, the consultants will develop recommendations for the final assessment report. Undoubtedly, some recommendations (hopefully, not too many) will be obvious ("you need greater cardiac surgery volume to cover your fixed costs"). Others will be insightful ("you can save $2 million annually by consolidating all your administrative offices into one off-site building"). Regardless, you must check them all for soundness before the consultants package them into a final report.

Your vetting of recommendations is essential because the recommendations are what you are paying for. Besides, recommendation development by consultants is as much an art as a science. You need to ensure that the recommendations are feasible and can generate the stated financial improvement. Vetting of recommendations also provides insight into the caliber of the firm. A consulting firm that recommends that you should build a new hospital, when you have no capital or means to raise it, should give you cause for concern. Vetting also is essential to the credibility of the final report-out sessions to stakeholders. A recommendation that the hospital recruit an additional ob/gyn physician to make a total of four—when the hospital already has five—is egregious and disastrous to the engagement.

Before you vet the recommendations, confirm that the leaders responsible for the affected areas have already vetted them. Remember: This is the last chance you and your senior team will have to express dissatisfaction with the consultants' work product. Once the consultants finalize and present their report, they have done their job. All that remains, unless there is an implementation phase, is for them to collect any outstanding fees from you.

Ensuring Clarity of the Assessment Report

Consulting firms commonly make their final report several hundred pages long. Most firms believe that, given the price of the engagement, clients expect a heavy tome in return. Some use these long and dense reports to mask weak work products. Even when the consultants' rationale is well intended, long, opaque reports detract from your ability to see whether you received value for money. Therefore, before the consulting firm finalizes its report, request an executive summary for your review. Your goal is to validate that the consulting firm fulfilled its agreement and that its recommendations are useful.

If at this late juncture you determine the work product is weak, refuse to pay unless the consultants agree to return to the trenches and improve their recommendations. Fight the temptation to accept the product and spin it to your organization as being better than it is. Many leaders tout horrible consulting engagements as amazing successes to avoid conflict with the consulting firm or stakeholders' criticism for buying shoddy work. Employees see through this spin, and at best, such reports end up on a shelf; at worst, the episode damages your credibility. It is better to be honest with the consultants. If you cannot make them improve their work product, be honest with employees.

Fortunately, rather than risk a poor sales reference, good consulting firms will either do more work to improve the report or give you a discount on the fees.

CONSULTANT'S TIP

The client has to be ready to hold their staff accountable for implementing changes that the consultant recommends. They must communicate this commitment to everyone prior to the engagement and then actually do that during the engagement.

—*Senior managing consultant, clinical*

ENGAGEMENT CHECKLIST

▶ Have you implemented a process to ensure the efficiency and security of the data request phase?

If you haven't, the symptoms will be clear: managers frustrated about voluminous, duplicative, and unclear requests; consultants frustrated about incomplete or conflicting data; finance department leaders anxious that managers are sending unverified data; compliance officers worried about privacy; and so on. If any of these symptoms occur, stop the data request and institute a data governance process. Better still, prevent the problem by instituting the governance process before launching the engagement.

▶ Have you reviewed the consultants' interview schedules and process?

You should have easy access to a list of the consultants' proposed interviews because most firms schedule interviews through one administrative assistant in the client's organization. To be certain that the list is complete, ask for the interview calendar from the consultants, too. Review the list to ascertain that the interviews are brief and the right consultants are interviewing the right people. In addition, require that the consultants create agendas and focused questions drawn from the data analysis.

▶ Do you know if the consultants will directly observe workflows?

Establish this expectation before you sign the agreement with the understanding that it may increase the cost of the engagement. Always ask for some, even if only limited, direct observation. It will improve the consultants' recommendations and your organization's acceptance of those recommendations.

▶ Have you reviewed a draft of the consultants' final report?

If the report is unworkably long, ask the firm to make it shorter and to start with a clear executive summary. If you find that the report's bulk is hiding a weak work product, ask the consulting firm to improve it.

REFERENCE

Oprah.com. 2011. "*The Oprah Winfrey Show* Finale." Published May 25. https://www.oprah.com/oprahshow/the-oprah-winfrey-show-finale_1/7.

CHAPTER 11

Causes of Failed Engagements

> **CONSULTANT'S TIP**
>
> The key success factors are communication of the project's goal early and often, support from every member of the C-suite, and agreement on how you will measure success.
>
> —*Managing director, nonlabor/supply chain consulting*

A COMMON CAUSE of failed engagements is a lack of support in the organization. Good consultants are wonderful at uncovering problems, making recommendations, and getting clients to agree to difficult recommendations—leading the horses to the water, so to speak. Great consultants can also be wonderful at implementing—getting the horses to drink. However, no consulting firm can complete an engagement without the support of the client's leaders and employees. This support is vital because consultants likely do not possess an established relationship with or a deep knowledge of the client's organization, know its political environment, or have the resources to implement recommended changes on their own. Clients must develop a culture of enthusiasm for change in their organization, preferably before hiring consultants and definitely before they leave. Successful engagements rely on this teamwork.

CASE 12

For a comprehensive consulting engagement at a 240-bed academic center in Florida, the consulting firm developed an initiative tracking document, or tracker, that it updated and presented weekly at a meeting of the hospital's senior leadership team. (Chapter 12 includes a detailed discussion about trackers.) The tracker did not quantify the dollars by initiative, but it did include timelines, responsible parties, and the overall target of $11 million in financial improvement. And it soon showed that two clinical initiatives had stalled.

The first ill-fated initiative called for the discharge of newborns for home phototherapy to avoid the cost of keeping mildly jaundiced babies an extra day or two in the hospital. This initiative stalled because most of the neonatologists refused to attend meetings to discuss the issue. Moreover, the lead neonatologist, who did attend the meetings, questioned the safety of relying on home phototherapy and declined to champion it with his colleagues. The second stalled initiative aimed to persuade interventional cardiologists to reduce the use of costly drug-eluting stents. The interventional cardiologists, all of whom were independent rather than employed, initially snubbed the consultants. Eventually, they attended a meeting to present a journal article showing that drug-eluting stents were a better option for many situations than cheaper, bare-metal stents. They also argued that they used an appropriate number of stents for the patients' diagnoses. Having delivered this message, they rejected any follow-up meetings.

The consultants sought help from the CEO who, in turn, asked the chief medical officer (CMO) to intercede. The

→

CASE 12
(continued)

CMO was unable to push either initiative forward.

At a tracker meeting later, the CEO asked how much the neonatology initiative would save the hospital annually. The answer was surprising. Given the low volume of babies qualifying for the home phototherapy and new case management costs to address the senior neonatologist's safety concerns, the annual savings would be only $25,000. Regarding the stents, the CEO asked for more evidence to support the interventional cardiologists' claims, and the consultants requested time to research the answer. The CMO did not advance either initiative, so the CEO decided to drop both.

LESSONS

1 Avoid spending time, effort, and political capital on initiatives that would generate low financial returns and have little impact on safety or quality. For the phototherapy initiative, the CEO should have required the consultants to track the targeted financial improvement. This would have revealed that the effort was not worth pursuing.

2 Make sure your consultants are qualified to tackle the initiatives they recommend. For the drug-eluting stents initiative, the clinical consulting team lacked the expertise and credibility to change the interventional cardiologists' practice patterns. Failure to identify weaknesses early will endanger the success of your engagement. Make sure your CMO is comfortable with the qualifications and experience of the consulting team members who intend to change physicians' practices. You should also ask the consultants how they intend to persuade physicians to accept changes.

3 Both the phototherapy and stent initiatives highlight a potential problem with the CMO. The CMO was ineffective in supporting the consultants' efforts. Indeed, as the engagement proceeded, other clinical initiatives stalled and the CMO was unable or unwilling to advance them. One way to ensure that your CMO is engaged and supportive is to ask the CMO to own the success of clinical initiatives. As part of this ownership, ask the CMO to present progress during the tracker reporting sessions. This will quickly expose any problems.

4 Engage your medical staff. Here, the refusal of some physicians to attend meetings was a symptom of disengagement. Before launching your consulting engagement, reflect on whether the physicians are engaged enough to partner with the consultants. If not, you have three options: (1) limit the initiatives to nonclinical areas as you work to improve physician engagement, (2) include clinical initiatives but take parallel steps to improve physician engagement, or (3) wait until you have improved physician engagement before you hire consultants. Your choice from the three options depends on how much runway you have and the degree of physician disengagement. My earlier book, *An Insider's Guide to Physician Engagement,* provides a systematic approach for attacking the issue (Agwunobi 2018).

WHEN INITIATIVES STALL

Implementation is hard, particularly when it comes to physician-related initiatives. This challenge can lead workgroups to become mired, unable to advance certain initiatives despite repeated meetings. Wheels can spin in place for four main reasons:

  1. *Analysis paralysis.* It is common, particularly when dealing with workgroups of physicians, for consultants to become captives in a never-ending cycle of data collection and

analysis. The physicians request data to substantiate the consultant's recommendations, findings in the new data lead to a request for more data, and so on. Eventually, the group loses momentum. Its members, busy with their day jobs, become distracted. The consultants become demoralized. Progress stalls.

Sometimes, the main cause of analysis paralysis is simply bad data. The consultants' data initially look impressive, but shortcomings appear as the workgroup drills deeper. Facilitation of workgroups is another important factor in analysis paralysis. An effective facilitator sets the expectation that data are only directional, which heads off gridlock and enables the group to plan and act. On the other hand, ineffective facilitators continue down rabbit holes after more data, even when the likely benefit of that data is marginal. In such situations, you may need to insert a new facilitator or simply direct the workgroup to move forward even as it collects more data.

CONSULTANT'S TIP

Clients should be forthcoming with their issues, open to change, and willing to make the tough decisions.

—*Director, integrated data management consultant*

---

2. *Stakeholder resistance.* Frequently, a workgroup spins its wheels because the staff opposes certain initiatives or the whole idea of consultants. The resistance may be passive-aggressive (missing meetings) or overt (challenging the consultants' understanding of the issues). Either way, progress on initiatives stops. A core role of the executive steering committee (ESC) is to help workgroups advance and to hold them accountable for missing targets, but you may need to intervene personally when employee resistance

leads to an impasse. You must first decide whether it is worth the effort to fix the situation. Sometimes, the resistance and rancor are so deep that it is better to disband the group and free the consultants to work on other initiatives. If implementation of the workgroup's initiatives is mission critical, preserve the group but insert a new leader or assume leadership yourself. Replacing problematic members is another potential intervention.

Resistance from senior executives is particularly damaging. This resistance can also be passive or overt. Employees, physicians, and other internal stakeholders will take cues from their leaders and progress will stall. You must address this directly and quickly. Options include coaching, reassigning, or replacing senior leaders who are not working for the success of the engagement.

3. *Wrong initiatives.* An initiative can stall because it is the wrong initiative. When this occurs, the consultants are typically at fault. Either their supporting data were inaccurate, they chose the initiative without realizing the juice wasn't worth the squeeze, or they didn't see that implementation would be impossible for political or other reasons. Jettison such initiatives before they delay the engagement and damage its credibility with employees. You may have to do so in the face of resistance from defensive consultants.

4. *Failure to work across departments.* Often, a workgroup associated with one department must work with another department on an initiative. In one such engagement, for example, a hospitalist workgroup aimed to decrease the number of unnecessary admissions. The hospitalists had to work with the emergency department (ED) to change the admissions process. One change called for the hospitalists rather than the ED physicians to admit patients. The hospitalists, however, had a poor relationship with the ED physicians and excluded them in the planning. Once

the ED physicians found out about the proposed change, they vehemently opposed it, effectively blocking any progress. To avoid such situations, the ESC must ensure that workgroups include all necessary stakeholders, even if only on an ad hoc basis. In this case, the ESC also could facilitate necessary changes to admitting privileges, hospital bylaws, and so forth.

CONSULTANT'S TIP

Both the quality and quantity of communications are critical. The best communication includes the rationale for the consulting engagement ("the house is on fire" works well) and promotes the expectations of the client management team, employees, and docs.

—*Managing director, clinical consulting*

ENGAGEMENT CHECKLIST

▶ Does your tracking document include all necessary metrics?

The tracking document should show the financial value of each initiative as well as the progress toward each initiative. If several stalls are attributable to one workgroup, investigate the workgroup's dynamics. Consider attending a meeting to evaluate the effectiveness of the facilitator, the degree of attendee resistance, and the status of data analysis. Attending workgroup meetings also allows you to set expectations and thank the attendees for their efforts.

▶ Is the clinical consulting team strong enough to engage in physician change management?

It is uneconomical for consulting firms to employ enough physician consultants to cover every major specialty. Still, you should understand how the firm intends to compensate for this lack of specialty-specific knowledge. You should also understand the consultants' change-management strategies. Ask the team for detailed examples of how they have previously changed physician practices.

▶ **Have you addressed resisters?**

This is particularly important when the resisters are members of your senior team. Face this problem proactively to prevent failure of the engagement, which will cause damage to your credibility as a leader.

REFERENCE

Agwunobi, A. C. 2018. *An Insider's Guide to Physician Engagement.* Chicago: Health Administration Press.

CHAPTER 12

Monitoring Success

CONSULTANT'S TIP

Identify the stakeholders. Put strong, supportive individuals in sponsor roles. Be honest about potential roadblocks, especially people who are not supportive, and be willing to move quickly to remove the roadblocks.

—*Senior managing consultant, physician practice management*

MONITORING THE SUCCESS of your consulting engagement is an imperative for both you and your consultants. This is particularly true for the implementation phase of engagements. That's when you typically pay a portion of the consultants' fees based on financial results, such as a 4:1 return on investment (ROI). Good consulting firms welcome monitoring. It prevents later squabbles about payment. In addition, when consultants can show that they delivered on their promises, their reputation and future sales prospects brighten.

HOW TO MEASURE IMPROVEMENT

There are three main ways to monitor success in an engagement: (1) tracking the progress of initiatives, (2) tracking the resulting financial improvement against projected improvement, and

(3) validating completion. These measurements are important because some initiatives will prove to be impracticable and others, even when implemented, may not lead to the promised financial improvement.

Tracking Progress

Without monitoring, you might waste a great deal of time and money before realizing that key initiatives are stalled and financial improvement proves to be elusive. At the end of the assessment phase, ask the consultants to provide a summary of their recommended initiatives. This list will also help you judge the quality of the assessment. If it comprises only a few items, or if many are vague, send it back to the consultants for improvement. This list should be the basis for a tracking document, or tracker, to monitor progress during the implementation. Trackers should always include the (1) name of each initiative with a brief description, (2) names of responsible leaders from the hospital and the consulting firm, (3) net financial savings or revenues by initiative, and (4) progress and estimated completion dates of each initiative.

A consultant–employee dyad should update and present the tracker to the executive steering committee (ESC) weekly or biweekly. Ideally, the consultant team leader updates the tracker, which the hospital employee—prepped by the consultant—presents to the ESC. Finally, the consultant fields any questions from ESC members. This format drives employee ownership and accountability, helps to ensure that hospital leaders will agree with the consultant's findings, and fosters a more collaborative meeting.

Checking Financial Improvement

In addition to monitoring the completion of initiatives at least biweekly, you and your organization's CFO should monitor the actual financial improvement, or *realization*, against the paper financial improvement on a monthly basis. For example, the consultants may document $800,000 in savings from a reduction in staffing. If this leads to an unanticipated $200,000 in overtime, you will only save $600,000. And if the reduction in staffing occurs in the ninth month of a yearlong engagement, you will only *realize* $150,000 in savings during that engagement. Thus, there are three reasons to append a realization schedule to an initiative tracker.

1. The estimated financial improvement from a completed initiative is just that: an estimate. You need to know the actual improvement.

2. Projected financial improvement might not occur right away. Results accrue over time. In fact, consulting firms often complete their engagements and depart months before all financial benefits are realized. So if a firm completes a departmental consolidation initiative that yields $120,000 in annual savings from the elimination of a director's position, the consultants will *report* $120,000 as your financial benefit. You, however, will *realize* only one-twelfth of that amount each month. The realization schedule will show this gain of $10,000 savings per month starting on the date the director departs, allowing you to compare how much you have saved in real dollars (e.g., $30,000 after three months) against the total projected financial benefit of $120,000.

3. A realization schedule is essential if you have negotiated an at-risk payment model for your consultants. Understandably, firms going at-risk cannot wait for you to receive the full financial benefit of all completed initiatives before you pay them. Nevertheless, knowing what you are realizing in real dollars enables you to adjust your rate of payment to match the bottom-line improvement and then to project whether the firm will actually hit the promised financial target.

Ask the consulting firm to develop the realization schedule, and be sure that the promised financial improvement is both reasonable and satisfies your ROI needs. Good consulting firms will be conservative by reducing the total anticipated improvement to reflect the chance of failure (i.e., probability adjusting). A good rule of thumb is to reduce the original identified improvement amount, or opportunity, by 50 percent with the assumption that half the initiatives will succeed and half will fail. For example, if an initial draft of a realization schedule shows the full financial improvement associated with completing all the initiatives to be $20 million, choose a target of $10 million. The consulting firm, from its experience, will know how to distribute realization of the $10 million across the duration of the engagement.

Behind each realization schedule and initiative tracker is the consulting firm's *benefit methodology* for arriving at estimated financial improvement from a completed initiative. You must understand and agree with this methodology—it underlies your promised financial improvement and the payments you will make under at-risk agreements. If consultants help you switch to a lower-cost orthopedic device, the benefit methodology would include the price of the original product during the baseline period minus the price of the new product multiplied by the volume of the original product during the baseline period. Armed with an understanding of the methodology's equation, you can sort out potential disagreements regarding the benefit to be credited to the consultants. One such disagreement can occur when patient volume after completion of the initiative is much lower than the baseline. The consultants delivered the promised savings per device, but the total savings fell short because of issues beyond the consultants' control.

Other benefit methodology calculations are more complex, as in reductions in average length of stay (ALOS). The CFO and the consultants must agree on the savings for an avoidable day in the hospital. For example, one West Coast public hospital's CFO asked the consultants to exclude the prison population from the calculation because the state department of corrections reimbursed at cost and the hospital did not control the wait times for secure transport. The CFO also asked the consultants to exclude the cost of all patients' supplies, because the hospital used most supplies during the early part of the admission rather than the last one to two days, subject to reduction. Other ALOS exclusions might include days associated with newborns and patients who died while in the hospital.

Your benefit methodology discussion with the consultants should also include how to avoid problems such as double-counting benefits. That might occur when the labor consulting team counts savings associated with flexing your nursing staff while the patient flow consulting team counts the same savings as associated with reducing your length of stay. The discussion should also establish how frequently (say, monthly or quarterly) the consulting firm should report on the realization of benefit for any initiative and how any benefit that your employees (rather than the consultants) implement should be reported and credited.

Validating Completion

In addition to agreeing on benefit methodology, you and the consulting firm must agree on the process for validating the completion of initiatives. This includes creating a benefit sign-off document and deciding who signs the document to formalize the completion of an initiative by the consultants.

Take the earlier example of the consolidation of two departments to save $120,000 by eliminating a director's job. It would be the responsibility of the vice president for the consolidated department to validate that the consolidation occurred, the net benefit (here, after payment of severance) is accurate, and the date the hospital will begin to realize actual dollar savings is correct.

CASE 13   The CEO of a 270-bed hospital in Florida hired a consulting firm for a comprehensive performance improvement engagement. The consultants spent a lot of time evaluating the hospital's robotic surgery program. The firm concluded that the hospital would save $500,000 annually from closing the program because only one surgeon used the da Vinci robot and most of her cases were gynecological procedures with low reimbursement. The consultants recommended closure.

In reviewing the initiative and its associated savings, the CEO expressed several concerns. First, the consultants overestimated the losses by not noting that the hospital had fully depreciated the robot. Second, the hospital recently had purchased a second robot and was heavily marketing the hospital's robotic capability. Third, the hospital's competitors had robots. Fourth, the CEO feared the hospital would be less successful in recruiting surgeons without a robot and might even lose its sole gynecological surgeon. The CEO declined to pursue the initiative.

LESSONS

1 From the outset of your engagement, communicate what is definitely out of scope. Many clients feel obliged to tell their consultants "nothing is off the table" or "there are no sacred cows." In truth, some things are off the table and some cows are sacred. Stipulating these upfront can prevent consultants from burning their time and wasting your money on fruitless endeavors.

2 Understand and agree with the methodology the consulting firm uses to arrive at its stated financial improvement for each initiative. This function is the responsibility of the CFO, but when the savings are large or the initiative is controversial, you should understand the methodology so that you can explain and defend it to stakeholders such as physicians or affected employees.

A realization schedule and a clear benefit methodology, followed by careful validation, are important. However, they will help only if you take the steps that are necessary and in your control to ensure real—not merely theoretical—financial improvement. Keep in mind that when the consulting firm identifies a way to reduce your hospital's ALOS, actual financial improvement may not result unless you follow through with marketing to fill the empty beds or implement a flex-staffing model for nurses to reduce staffing costs. If the consultants help you replace a manual process with an electronic one that can cut staffing costs, you will only realize those savings if you actually reduce the staff. It is your job to fill the beds, reallocate nurses when ALOS decreases, or eliminate positions. Of course, you may still decide to pursue such initiatives solely for the quality and safety benefits, but if you are at fault for not realizing the financial improvement, the consulting firm may still expect you to validate the financial benefit and pay accordingly.

CONSULTANT'S TIP

From a revenue cycle perspective, our clients achieve faster results when the CEO and CFO identify us as the drivers, on their behalf, of the engagement from the top down. A resistant director in the business office can make it difficult to implement what we know is a proven methodology to increase cash, reduce days for collection of accounts receivable, and reduce claim denials.

—*Managing consultant, revenue cycle*

ENGAGEMENT CHECKLIST

▶ **Have you informed the consulting firm of the issues that are out of scope?**

You might not want to cut back on a recently expanded service. Maybe you want to continue a money-losing clinic for mission purposes. Perhaps political considerations prevent you from eliminating certain positions. Regardless of the reason, tell the consultants about any sacred cows upfront. This will prevent them from wasting resources and generating unnecessary turmoil in the organization.

▶ **Have you created an initiative-tracking document to monitor progress?**

The key metrics in a consulting engagement include the initiatives' dollar values and timelines for completion. Common failings of these trackers occur when the initiatives are vague, such as those simply labeled "implement staffing reductions," or when the dollars are not quantified. Make yours specific, as in this example: "Consolidate two medical director positions in the cancer center for savings of $360,000."

▶ Have you and the consulting firm agreed on a realization schedule?

Once you have agreed on the realization schedule, match your at-risk payments to the schedule. For example, if the realization schedule shows more dollars saved in the second half of a one-year engagement, your scheduled payments to the consulting firm should be less in the first half of the year and more in the second half.

▶ Have you and the consulting firm agreed on the benefit methodology?

Take an initiative-by-initiative approach to establishing the benefit methodology as soon as you receive the consulting firm's list of recommendations. Agreeing on benefit methodologies can be time consuming, so there is no point to hashing out benefit methodologies to reduce personnel if staffing reductions are out of scope.

CHAPTER 13

Ensuring Sustainability

> **CONSULTANT'S TIP**
>
> Clients should first identify the appropriate internal people
> to engage with consultants during the engagement,
> be champions of the engagement in the organization,
> and ultimately commit to maintaining success after the
> consultants leave.
>
> —*Managing consultant, integrated data management*

UNHAPPILY, CONSULTING ENGAGEMENTS frequently go from
backslapping to back to Square One in just a few years. You can
prevent this fate for your engagement. The first step is to view sustainability as the responsibility of your organization, not the consulting
firm. Every consulting firm will swear it excels at ensuring sustainability, and the good ones will follow through with efforts such as
training your employees and leaving behind tools. The truth, however,
is that training and tools from consulting firms alone are inadequate.

DRIVERS OF EFFECTIVE CHANGE

The most important drivers of sustainability are changes that only
leaders of the hospitals themselves can effect. The following are
descriptions of those drivers.

- *Change organizational structure.* When you change organizational structure, you ensure that a new process cannot backslide. The structure change hardwires the improvement. For example, in one engagement, the consultants created a physician-adviser position whose role was to prevent and respond to denials from insurance plans. This new position reported to the associate vice president of case management who, in turn, reported to the chief nursing officer. Historically, the chief medical officer (CMO) performed this function, but because of his busy schedule, denials management was suboptimal. The consultants could have had the new position report to the CMO, but they knew the reporting line to case management would add synergies and sharpen the function. The new position succeeded in improving denials management. Although consultants can recommend such organizational changes, the leader has to be willing to implement them—even in the face of organizational politics and resistance.
- *Replace ineffective leaders.* One of the most effective ways to achieve sustainability is to replace ineffective leaders. Consulting engagements frequently uncover leaders who resist change or lack the competence or energy to implement change. Try coaching such leaders, but if that fails, replace them. Leaving ineffective leaders in place will erode your consulting engagement gains.
- *Perpetuate new routines.* After the end of an engagement, continue routines that the consultants started. In one example of this driver, consultants set up a multidisciplinary vacancy review committee that met biweekly to review all new positions. This routine helped the organization achieve significant labor cost savings from attrition. After the consultants departed, the CEO continued the committee meetings. Three years later, the committee still functioned, helping the

organization to maintain and even deepen its savings. In another organization, consultants used a portion of the hospital's weekly senior executive team meeting as the executive steering committee (ESC) meeting. After the engagement, the CEO continued this routine but dedicated the ESC portion to seeing that the executives were sustaining and even expanding the consultants' initiatives. The hospital sustained its consulting gains, and the frequent meetings engendered a culture of greater operational and financial discipline.

CONSULTANT'S TIP

Clients can get the best out of a consulting engagement by first explaining the mission of the engagement as well as the current state of the organization. As an example: "We are losing $1 million a month, and it is imperative for everyone to help support the initiatives to help us improve the financial state of the system."

—*Managing consultant, nonlabor/supply chain*

To maintain new routines after the engagement, you and the consulting firm should create them with permanency in mind. This includes setting the expectation with both your leaders and employees that the routines will outlive the consulting engagement. It also includes making the routines convenient. When frequent meetings are involved, be sure to make them brief and piggyback them with existing meetings when possible.

- *Create a sustainability culture.* Your goal for a comprehensive performance improvement consulting engagement should go beyond improving operations and finances. It should be to transform your organization's culture. The first step toward this goal is to weave the consultants into the fabric of your organization. Make the consultants an extension of your leaders and employees. In this way, the consultants' culture—making decisions according to data, embracing and driving change, facing tough decisions, holding people accountable, and carrying a bias toward action—diffuses throughout your organization. After the consultants leave, start new routines that further incorporate the consultants' culture. For example, after one engagement, the CEO started biweekly financial improvement project sessions where the senior executives set new financial improvement goals beyond those that the consultants set and then identified initiatives to meet those goals. This routine instilled a culture of efficiency, data-based decision-making, and accountability while sustaining prior consulting gains.

CASE 14

A reversal of financial improvement following a consulting engagement occurred between 2004 and 2010 at Jackson Health System (JHS), a public hospital system in Florida. JHS included a flagship hospital with more than 1,550 beds, a children's hospital, 12 primary care centers, and several associated healthcare organizations. In March 2004, JHS faced serious financial difficulty. It had experienced a net income loss of $47 million in fiscal year 2003, and $85 million in FY 2004. The system was projecting a loss of $140 million for 2005 and had less than 30 days cash on hand. JHS engaged a consulting firm to assist with a comprehensive financial turnaround effort that the hospital and the firm branded "reCreate Jackson" (O'Quinn and Mulqueen 2007).

→

CASE 14
(continued)

The multiyear effort took a great deal of work with up to 120 consultants at its peak. In 2007, the firm and hospital leaders wrote a case study describing their approach to solving the interdependent problems of the large and complex organization. They noted the many focal points, including revenue cycle, staff productivity, overtime and use of agencies, senior management overhead, costs of the academic mission, and supply and service expenses (O'Quinn and Mulqueen 2007). The engagement was a success. By 2005, the consultants had reversed JHS's losses and the system posted a $10 million profit. JHS also went on to post a positive margin in 2006 (O'Quinn and Mulqueen 2007). Unfortunately, deep financial trouble returned, and JHS posted a $244 million loss in 2010 (Dorschner 2010). In response, leadership announced steep cuts in staffing, pay, and benefits as parts of another turnaround effort (Chang 2016).

LESSONS

1 Multiple cost and revenue factors can contribute to the erosion of consulting gains. Sustainability goes beyond maintaining the consultant-led changes. It also includes addressing any external financial stressors, such as strong competitors, a worsening payer mix, or funding cuts that contributed to the original need for an engagement. In other words, even when an engagement is successful and the consulting gains stick, the organization's finances may slip backward because of factors outside the scope of the engagement. An efficacious consulting engagement at least will provide breathing room to address these challenges.

2 Do not wait until the end of your engagement to implement sustainability measures. At the engagement's onset, require the consulting firm to provide any necessary tools and training. Throughout the engagement, implement the organizational structure changes and other changes for long-term sustainability.

STRATEGIES FOR SUSTAINABILITY

As noted earlier, good consulting firms try to establish sustainability. Not all, however, bake sustainability elements into the project. All too often, consultants and clients alike consider sustainability efforts to be the final additions to an engagement—the icing on the cake rather than the primary ingredients, or strategies, they should start with. In fact, there are proven strategies for you and your consultants to employ that can yield enduring success.

- *Knowledge transfer.* It would be great if your consultants could simply upload their knowledge directly to your employees, but they can't. Consultants and employees alike are generally too busy for extensive training sessions, and consultants have little financial incentive to spend a lot of time teaching. One solution is for the consultants to provide targeted training. For example, at one hospital, consultants recommended that ob/gyn physicians use an inexpensive medication for cervical ripening during induction of labor in place of the costlier drug they were using. The targeted training included inviting a well-respected expert from another university to present to the hospital's physicians. Other examples include labor consultants training employees on using a staffing grid, nonlabor/supply chain consultants training academic medical center residents on a new floor stock policy and food formulary, and revenue cycle consultants training preregistration staff on credit card handling procedures.

- *Policy changes.* Consultant-led training is essential for sustainability but insufficient on its own. Consultants also must recommend and drive changes in policies. Policy changes, like organizational structure changes, can hardwire any improvements. In the ob/gyn initiative example, consultants worked with the pharmacy and therapeutics committee to remove the more expensive medication from the hospital formulary. This change also involved working with the physicians to modify the existing cervical ripening and induction order set. As a rule, organizations must communicate policy changes widely for them to be effective.

- *Tools.* Consultants also sustain change by introducing new tools. For example, in one hospital a revenue cycle consulting team introduced a patient-estimation tool to the dermatology department staff. This software enabled the staff to give new patients a written cost estimate of services. This, in turn, increased the likelihood that patients would pay and improved patient satisfaction.

It should be noted that consulting firms might not own all the tools that their clients need. Consultants frequently ask clients to purchase tools from third parties. For clinical cost improvement initiatives, the consultants might ask clients to buy a license for a software and classification system that categorizes patients into manageable clinical groups. Major requests would include the purchase of an electronic health record system or a cost-accounting system. If you can't afford third-party tools, work with the consulting firm to create homegrown tools that will ensure sustainability. Even when consulting firms own the tools, you should not assume that they will leave them behind. For example, one consulting firm owned a cutting-edge proprietary data analysis software that it used during an engagement. The client's employees loved the tool, and they were dismayed to learn at the end of the engagement that the firm didn't consider it a "leave behind." The client negotiated access to the software, hosted by the consulting firm, after the engagement ended.

- *Monitor sustainability.* Consider asking the consulting firm to monitor sustainability beyond the end of the engagement. For example, in one engagement, the CEO asked the consulting firm to monitor sustainability at monthly intervals for a year after the engagement. The consulting team leaders accomplished this by calling into a monthly meeting of the client's vice presidents and directors to review dashboards, give advice, and answer questions. Consulting team leaders traveled to the hospital every three months to attend the meeting in person.

When negotiating the price of the engagement, consider asking for a postengagement maintenance period as a free or low-cost add-on. This is similar to asking for a period of free maintenance when negotiating the price of a car. The consulting firm may want to charge you more or may balk completely if you wait until the end of the engagement to ask.

CONSULTANT'S TIP

Communicate the engagement and its core objectives early and often to ensure that the engagement takes the highest (or nearly highest) priority for everyone at the organization. Drive accountability for adoption and engagement of analytics, metrics, and any complementary performance improvement tools.

—*Senior management consultant, integrated data management*

ENGAGEMENT CHECKLIST

▶ **Have you developed a strategy to address financial stressors outside the scope of your engagement?**

Plan well ahead for the postengagement period. The consulting gains will be short-lived if preexisting challenges such as decreasing reimbursement, increasing competition, or declining patient volumes remain. Consider whether you need strategic consulting assistance to address such challenges. Many consulting firms can provide this along with the management consulting services.

▶ **Have you asked what specific tools and training the consulting firm will provide?**

Do not be satisfied with generic answers such as "we train the trainers," or "we leave behind tools." Ask about specific training and decide whether the training is efficient and essential. In addition, ascertain the tools that the consultants will leave behind. Request that they leave the tools that they used during the engagement, and ask what you might need to purchase to supplement the firm's toolbox.

▶ **Are you hardwiring changes?**

Whenever the consultants implement a change, consider whether it calls for a change in policy, organizational structure, or leadership to hardwire it into your hospital's operations. Continually evaluate the routines initiated by the consultants to identify those that you will want to prolong after they depart. In addition, create new postengagement routines to maintain financial and operational discipline.

▶ **Have you asked the consultants for postengagement monitoring?**

Consider asking the consultants to monitor their work and provide guidance for some period after the engagement ends. This commitment will improve your chances of sustaining the gains and will motivate the consultants to focus on sustainability during the engagement. The consultants can accomplish this efficiently by means of teleconferencing rather than in-person meetings.

REFERENCES

Chang, D. 2016. "On Brink of Disaster, Jackson Turns Profitable Thanks to Visionary CEO." *Miami Herald.* (updated April 30, 2016).

Dorschner, J. 2010. "$244 Deficit: Jackson Health System 'A Colossal Mess' Says Miami-Dade Grand Jury." *Palm Beach Post.* August 6, 2010 (updated April 1, 2012).

O'Quinn, M., and K. C. Mulqueen. 2007. "ReCreate Jackson: A Turnaround Tale." *Healthcare Financial Management* 61 (7): 82–8.

About the Author

ANDREW C. AGWUNOBI, MD, is CEO and executive vice president for health affairs at UConn Health, the University of Connecticut's billion-dollar academic health system. Before joining UConn Health, Dr. Agwunobi—a pediatrician with a master's degree in business administration from the Stanford Graduate School of Business— served as managing director and a coleader of the Berkeley Research Group (BRG) healthcare performance improvement consulting practice. Before joining BRG, Dr. Agwunobi served as CEO of Providence Healthcare, a five-hospital system in Spokane, Washington. He earlier held the positions of president and CEO of Grady Health System in Atlanta, Georgia; president and CEO of Tenet South Fulton Hospital in East Point, Georgia; chief operating officer of the 14-hospital St. Joseph Health System in California; and secretary of the Florida Agency for Health Care Administration, responsible for the state's $16 billion healthcare administration budget.

Tenet Healthcare awarded Dr. Agwunobi its CEO Circle of Excellence Award in 2003. *Georgia Trend* magazine named him one of the 100 Most Influential Georgians in 2005, and *Modern Healthcare* magazine named him one of the nation's 50 Most Powerful Physician Executives in Healthcare in 2007. Other honors include CEO of the Year, Trailblazer category (Atlanta Business League, 2005), Most Influential Atlantans (*Atlanta Business Chronicle,* 2005), Speaker and Citizen of the Year (Atlanta Peachtree Rotary, 2004) and Agent of Change Award (*Catalyst* magazine, 2002).

Dr. Agwunobi served on the board of directors of Gonzaga University, with an appointment to the adjunct faculty in the business school. Dr. Agwunobi's previous book, *An Insider's Guide to Physician Engagement*, was published in 2018 by Health Administration Press.